Essential Skills

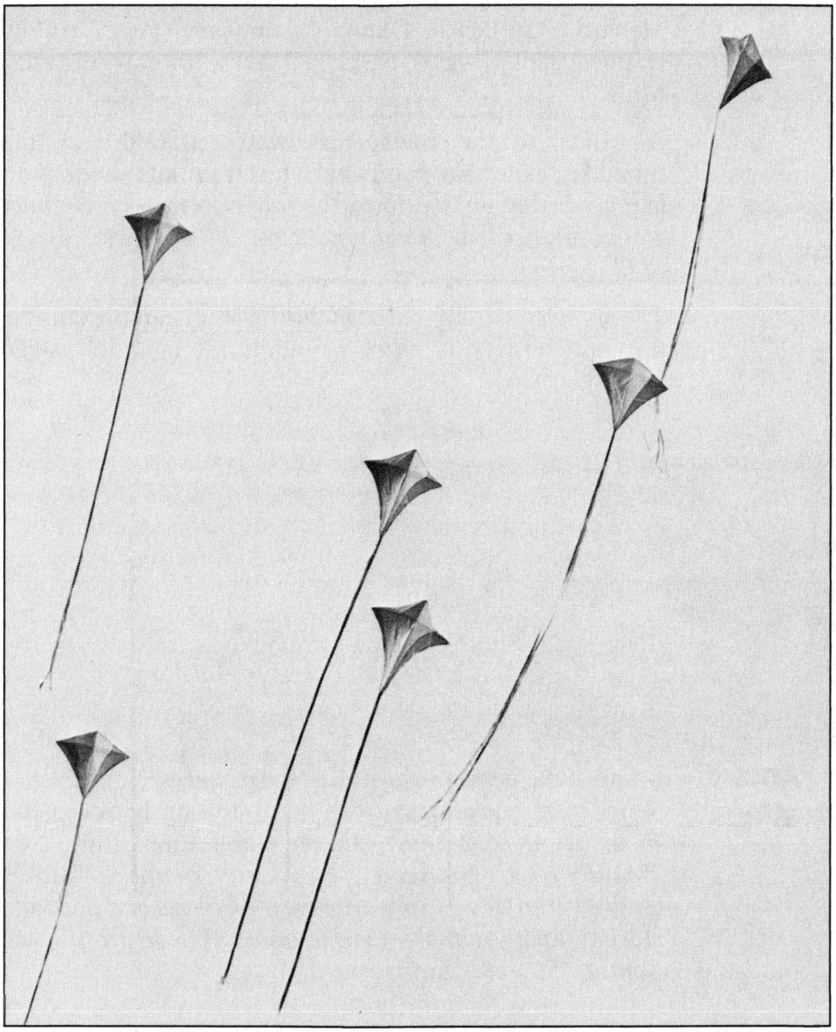

Revised Edition

About the Cover

The breeze was fresh this bright day in May, and gaily-colored kites appeared like spring swallows, darting across the blue sky over Rhode Island's Narragansett Bay. Photographer Tony Botelho was there to capture on film the kite-flights of Christy Menard, Art Pelosi, Danny Champagne, Peggy Hulsey, John Rathjen, Jack Christie, Stephen Jencks, Marion Alig and Megen Mills.

A salute to the rowboaters who retrieved the "diamond-spinnaker" kite that got away! The errant kite shook in the wind like a wet dog and rejoined the others in the sky, completing the composition of the photograph on the covers of the *Essential Skills Series*.

The six kites symbolize the higher levels of comprehension gained through mastery of skills from the six essential categories of comprehension.

About the Illustrations

Many of the pictures illustrating the passages in the *Essential Skills Series* were reproduced from the following books in the *Dover Pictorial Archive Series*, Dover Publications, Inc., New York: *Treasury of Art Nouveau, Design and Ornament*, Carol Belanger Grafton; *Harter's Picture Archive for Collage and Illustration*, Jim Harter; and *Animals: A Pictorial Archive from Nineteenth-Century Sources*, Jim Harter.

Other illustrations are by Howard Lewis and Thomas Ewing Malloy.

Essential Skills Series

Essential Skills Book 5

Walter Pauk, Ph.D.
Director, Reading Research Center
Cornell University

Revised Edition

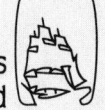

Jamestown Publishers
Providence, Rhode Island

Essential Skills Series
No. 305, Book 5

Copyright © 1982 by Jamestown Publishers, Inc.

All rights reserved. The contents of this book are protected by the United States Copyright Law. It is illegal to copy or reproduce any pages or parts of any pages. Address all inquiries to Editor, Jamestown Publishers, Post Office Box 9168, Providence, Rhode Island 02940.

Cover Design by Deborah Hulsey Christie, adapted from the Original Design by Stephen R. Anthony

Text Design by Deborah Hulsey Christie

Printed in the United States of America

9 10 11 12 13 PO 96 95 94 93 92

ISBN 0-89061-224-2

Preface

Practice Makes Perfect

Why do some students shoot baskets over and over again and others skate and reskate the same routine? These beginners know that practice makes perfect. Not only do beginners know this, but pros do too. For what other reason do they work at baseball and football week after week before the opening dates?

Value of Practice

The pros know the value of practice, but they also know the value of something else. They know that practice without *instruction* and *guidance* does not automatically lead to improvement. That's why they have the best coaches that money can buy.

And so it is with developing the skills of reading. There must be the right kind of practicing and the right kind of coaching.

First, a word about practice. In this book the right kind of practice is provided by twenty-five highly interesting and carefully selected passages. Here is material enough on which to grow and keep growing.

Value of Coaching

Now about coaching! Good coaching takes the form of instruction and guidance. In this book the instruction is straightforward and uncomplicated. It puts you directly on the right track, and better still, you are kept on the right track by two unusual systems of guidance. The first system is the uniquely designed, six-way question format which makes sure that every ounce of practice is directed toward improvement. Nothing is wasted!

Diagnostic Chart

The second system of guidance is the Diagnostic Chart. This chart is no ordinary gimmick. In truth, it provides the most dignified form of diagnosis and guidance yet devised. It provides instantaneous and continuous diagnosis and gentle but certain self-guidance. It yields information directly to the student. This form of self-guidance leads to the goal of all education: the goal of self-teaching.

Acknowledgments

Now, I want to make some acknowledgments, especially to the students who were the guinea pigs. Afterwards I told them so, but they said, "We didn't mind even then. And now that it is over, we're all the happier because we know how much we've learned." But what the students did not know was how much I learned from them. For this I thank them all, class after class.

I direct especial thanks to Linda Browning, Anita DuBose, and Karen Duddy for handling the almost countless number of selections, writing and refining the questions and making sure that the series kept moving: all, a most demanding task.

Finally, I am most grateful to authors, editors and publishers who have generously given permission to quote and reprint in this book from works written and published by them. The books quoted in the text and used as sources of reading extracts are listed in the back of the book.

Walter Pauk

Contents

To the Instructor   **8**
To the Student   **11**
    Understanding the Six Essential Skills   **11**
    Answering the Main Idea Question   **17**
    Getting the Most Out of This Book   **19**
Passages and Questions   **23**
Answer Key   **100**
Diagnostic Chart   **102**
Progress Graph   **103**
Classroom Management System   **106**

To the Instructor

Selection of Passages

All of us believe in this truism: to learn to read, a person must read. But, placing a book in front of a student won't automatically promote reading.

This last sentence brings up another truism: you can lead a horse to water, but you can't make it drink. To tempt a horse, the water must be clear, cool and clean.

To tempt the student, the passages must be genuinely fascinating. Knowing this, we packed each book with twenty-five "I can't put the book down" type of passages.

Each passage had to meet at least the following criteria: *high interest level, appropriate readability level* and *factual accuracy of contents*. High interest was assured by choosing passages from popular magazines that appeal to a wide range of readers. The readability level of each passage was assessed by applying Dr. Edward B. Fry's *Formula for Estimating Readability,* thus enabling the arrangement of passages on a single grade level within each book. The factual accuracy of the passages is high because they were written by professional writers whose works are recognized and respected.

The Great Value of Questions

Dr. Mortimer J. Adler says that the overall secret for improving one's reading can be boiled down to knowing how to keep awake while reading. He means more than keeping one's eyes open. He means keeping one's mind open and active.

One sure-fire way to do this is to keep trying to answer questions while reading. Questions not only keep one's mind awake, but also keep the mind active, not letting it get flabby. Here's a good story that makes the same point.

> To keep their fish alive for the fresh-fish markets, the owners of fishing boats used a water-filled floating tank. The fish remained alive all right, but they were never firm, always flabby. One captain, however, always brought back firm, fresh, active fish. His fish always received a higher price.

One day he revealed his secret: "You see," he said, "for every hundred herrings I put into my tank, I put in one catfish. It is true that the catfish eat five or six of the herrings on the trip back to port, but the catfish keep the rest alert and constantly active. That's why my herring arrive in beautiful condition."

The work of the catfish, in this book, is done by the six essential questions (subject matter, supporting details, conclusion, clarifying devices, vocabulary in context, and main idea). These questions keep the minds of students alert, active and in beautiful condition.

The main idea questions in this book are not the usual multiple-choice variety. Given four statements, the students are asked to recognize the main idea of the passage. They also tell why each of the other three does not express the main idea; the students identify one statement as too narrow, one as too broad and one as merely a detail.

By asking these six types of questions in each passage, students quickly learn to read with a questioning and anticipating attitude. This attitude, necessary for high comprehension, is easily transferred to other material such as the textbook.

The Diagnostic Chart

Those who used the first edition of these books had high praise for the Diagnostic Chart. In sum, this is what they said.

> The Diagnostic Chart is truly ingenious because it is, in fact, a self-diagnosing instrument. The Chart instantly, simply and continually shows students their strengths and weaknesses.

Here is how the Chart works. The six questions for each passage are always in the same order. For example, the question designed to teach the skill of making *conclusions* is always in the number three position, and the question designed to teach the skill of identifying *clarifying devices* is always in the number four position, and so forth. This innovation of keeping the questions in order sets the stage for the smooth functioning of the Chart.

The Chart works automatically when the letters of the answers are placed in the spaces on the Chart. Even after completing one passage, the Chart will reveal the type or types of questions answered correctly as well as the types answered incorrectly. But more important, the Chart will identify the types of questions missed consistently. More persuasive identification is possible after three or more passages have been completed. By then, a pattern can be observed. For example, if the answers to question number three (making conclusions) are incorrect for all three passages, or on three out of four, then this weakness shows up automatically.

Once a weakness is revealed, instruct the students to take the following steps: First, turn back to the instructional pages to study the section in which the topic is discussed. Second, go back to read again the questions in that particular category that were missed; then, with the correct answers in mind, read the entire passage again, trying to see how the author developed the answers to the questions. Third, on succeeding passages, put forth extra effort to answer correctly the questions in that particular category. Fourth, if the difficulty still persists, arrange for a conference with the instructor.

To the Student

Understanding the Six Essential Skills

How do readers get the meaning from written words? To get meaning, readers need to know at least six essential skills.

1. Subject Matter — Readers need to know how to concentrate or focus on the writing. This helps them learn what the writing is about.
2. Main Idea — Readers need to know how to grasp the main idea or point of the writing.
3. Supporting Details — Readers need to be able to connect supporting details to the ideas.
4. Conclusions — Readers should be able to come to conclusions or guess endings based on the ideas.
5. Clarifying Devices — Readers should be able to note the writer's methods of making the points clear and alive.
6. Vocabulary in Context — Readers must know what the words in the writing mean.

Let's take a closer look at these six skills.

Concentration/ Subject Matter

One thing readers often say is, "I can't concentrate!" But there is a sure, fast cure. There is no better way to gain concentration when reading than this. Read the first few lines. Then ask yourself these questions: "What is this passage about?" "What is the subject matter?"

If you don't ask these questions, here's what may happen. Your eyes will move across the lines of print. Yet your mind will be thinking of other things.

But if you ask the questions, you will most likely get an answer, thus achieving concentration. Let's see if this method works. Here are the first lines of a passage:

> Wood ducks are the most beautiful ducks in North America. Once they were rare. Now — if you have sharp eyes and can keep quiet — you might see them in almost any woodland along streams and ponds.

After reading this, you can see that the author will talk about the wood duck. Now that your mind is on the trail, the chances are good it will follow the author's idea line by line. Thus, you will *concentrate* on the building of the subject matter.

Let's try the method again. Here are a few lines from another passage:

> Of all the little animals in the world, the Columbian ground squirrel is one of the liveliest and friendliest. It is nicknamed "picket pin." This is because it sits as stiff and straight as a stake in the ground.

Again, you most likely had no trouble picking out the subject. It is the Columbian ground squirrel.

Main Idea Once the subject matter has been grasped, it is time for the next question. Ask yourself, "What is the author's main idea?" "What point is the passage trying to make?"

With such questions in mind, you can be sure an answer will often pop up. But when no questions are asked, all things seem the same. Nothing stands out. The reader will not see the point of the passage.

Let's look at another passage. This time we will find the main idea.

> Wood ducks never nest on the ground as most ducks do, but in a big hole in a tree. Trees with big holes in them are hard to find.

You don't have the full passage to read, so I will tell you the answer. The main point is that with fewer and fewer old, dead trees with big holes in them, we will have fewer and fewer wood ducks.

Thus, when questions are asked, the reader is acting upon the content. Reading becomes a two-way street with both reader and writer engaged. In a sense, the reader talks with the author. So the passage comes to life. Reading then is a joy.

Supporting Details

Do we like details? Of course we do. In long pieces of writing, main ideas are like the bones. They are the skeleton of the writing. The details are the flesh. They give the writing fullness and life.

Details are used to support the main ideas. So the term *supporting details* fits well. These supporting details come in many forms. The most common forms are examples, definitions, comparisons, contrasts, repetitions and descriptions.

The author of "The Wood Duck" lets us know that the passage is about wood ducks. Next, the author makes sure we learn that the point is that without trees with holes, the wood duck will not nest. Thus, there would be fewer wood ducks.

Now that we are involved in this problem, the author gives us details on how we can provide trees with holes in them. The author *describes* how we can build a wood duck nesting box. Here's the excerpt:

> Why don't you and your parents put up a wood duck nesting box right now? It would be about two feet (about .61 meters) high and ten inches (about 25.4 centimeters) square. Make the entry hole about four inches (about 10.2 centimeters) across. Use rough lumber on the inside, so the ducklings can climb up the sides to the hole. Put wood shavings on the bottom. In these the duck will lay her eggs. To keep her eggs warm, she covers them with her own feathers. If you can't find a tree near the water, you will need a post. Place the box ten to thirty feet (about 3.1 to 9.1 meters) high.

You can see in the above passage how important details are in telling a story. Details let the reader see what's going on. They paint a vivid picture of the action. They may tell how to do something. They may tell how something happened.

In long passages there will also be sub-ideas. It is important to be careful not to mistake a sub-idea for a main idea. Sub-ideas are broader than details. But sub-ideas are still not the main point. The main idea has to do with the whole passage. The sub-idea has to do with just part of it. Note that in the next sample, the sub-idea is about the food that wood ducks eat. The whole passage is not about food. Thus, food is *not* the main idea. For the most part, you will see that a sub-idea takes the space of one paragraph. Often, the topic sentence of the paragraph is a statement of a sub-idea.

The following excerpts show how the author groups and structures supporting details around the sub-ideas that are stated in topic sentences. A sub-idea will hold a group of details together.

> Wood ducks eat acorns and all kinds of nuts. Their stomachs (or gizzards) have strong muscles. They can break the hardest nuts, some that you could barely crack with a hammer, in their stomachs. Wood ducks like berries, duckweed and insects. But best of all they like to eat spiders. That's ice cream to them.

The topic sentence is the first sentence. It states that the sub-idea is the foods wood ducks eat. Next, the author describes how the newly hatched ducklings get down to the ground from the nest.

Here are more details grouped around a sub-idea.

> Sometimes they nest in holes up in trees that are twice as high as a flagpole. Just think, the baby ducklings must jump to the ground the day they hatch. They don't get hurt, though, because they're light, like little puffs of cotton. The mother stands at the foot of the tree and calls and calls. The ducklings peek out of the hole. Then, like little paratroopers, they jump quickly, one right after the other, to join their mother. She must then hurry them to the pond where they're safe.

Thus, one of the main jobs of *supporting details* is to give some fullness to the passage. The passage would be just a boring, skimpy statement of the main idea with its bare-boned sub-ideas if not for details. The details give the passage life.

Conclusion The reader will move through a passage, grasping the main and sub-ideas and their details. It is then common for the reader to start to guess a conclusion or ending to the story. Such guesses are part of the sport of reading. Often, the author gives the reader an ending. In such a case, the joy of reading lies in the fact that the reader finds out the guess was right. But the ending may not be given. The reader then will try to guess the ending that is hinted by the author.

The conclusion from the excerpts just read about the wood duck is in having the reader see the pleasure of observing a wood duck. The final sentence is this:

> If you're lucky, though, and if your (duck) house is in place before the ice melts, you will have a wood duck family in the summer.

In a passage called "From Pond to Prairie," the author has this conclusion:

> Finally, there is no longer much open water. The pond has disappeared. Depending on the kinds of plants that have filled it, the pond may be called a bog or a marsh. As changes continue for many more years, the bog may become a forest.

The skillful reader is like a detective. This reader follows the story, always thinking, "Where is the author leading me?" "What's the final point?" "What's the conclusion?" And the reader, like a detective, must try to guess the conclusion, changing the guess if necessary as the story unfolds.

Clarifying Devices The author uses clarifying devices to make the points in the story clear and alive. In a sense, the *topic sentence* may be thought of as a clarifying device. It is often placed at the start of a paragraph. In this way, the author gives the reader a quick point of focus.

The point of the passage becomes clear after reading it.

But more often, by clarifying devices, we mean the literary devices in the passage. These are words or phrases which keep the ideas, sub-ideas and details in clear focus and in order.

Authors use literary devices to make details clear and interesting. An example of a device is the *metaphor,* as in "But best of all they like to eat spiders. *That's ice cream to them.*"

One more literary device is the *simile.* "*Like little paratroopers,* they (the ducklings) jump quickly, one right after the other, to join their mother," is a simile. The simile helps the reader imagine a vivid scene. It brings to the mind of the reader something known — paratroopers. Then it compares the known idea to the ducklings' jump from their nest to make a fresh, new idea. It is fun to imagine the little ducks copying real paratroopers jumping from a plane.

Besides metaphors and similes, other *clarifying devices* are organizational patterns. One common pattern is to unfold the events in the order of time. Thus, one thing happens first and then another and another, and so forth.

The time pattern orders the event. The event may take place in the span of five minutes. It may last hundreds of years. A time pattern may be used to relate the habits of an animal from its birth to its death.

You should learn to find these literary devices. They help you to understand the passage and speed your reading.

Vocabulary in Context

A reader who does not know what the author's words mean may not understand the passage. A reader should look up in the dictionary the unknown words.

Also a reader may understand only the general meaning of the word. But sometimes a more *exact* meaning is needed to grasp the passage fully. A reader who places a general meaning on a word may end up with a blurred picture of the idea. An exact meaning will give the reader a full and clear picture.

For instance, in the next excerpt are two common words that many people feel they already know. Thus, they don't see the need to look them up in the dictionary. But few people know the exact meaning of these words.

> Depending on the kinds of plants that have filled it, the pond may be called a *bog* or a *marsh*.

Do you know the difference between a bog and a marsh? Is there a difference? If so, what is it? How would your mental picture change if you knew?

Looking up words for their exact meanings is rewarding. A precise vocabulary leads to true understanding.

You may find it troublesome to look up words you feel you already know. But you should get into this habit to improve your reading. Of course, words you do not know must always be looked up. You would most likely need a dictionary for these words:

> Nothing could appear more *benign* than a field aglow with daisies, goldenrod and Queen Anne's lace.
>
> *Sphinxlike,* it crouches among the flowers until the desired insect wanders within reach.

The dictionary is like a stock market. Here you exchange fuzzy meanings for exact meanings. You get new meanings for unknown words. All this is at no cost. It takes just a flip of your finger.

Answering the Main Idea Question

To be able to find the main idea of the things you read is important. It is one of the best reading skills you can learn. The main idea questions in this book are not the ones you've seen where you pick just the right answer. Instead, each main idea question is made up of four statements. Two of the statements refer to just parts of the passage. One of these is a *detail*. It states a point. But that point has little to do with the passage as a whole. The next statement is *too narrow*. It tells more than the detail statement. Still, it's too specific to tell about the main point of the passage. The "too narrow" statement is often a sub-idea.

The last two statements deal with the whole passage. One is *too broad*. It is too general and too vague to be a good main idea statement. The final statement is the *main idea*. It tells *who* or *what* the point of the passage is. The main idea statement answers the question *does what?* or *is what?* also.

Read the sample passage below. Then follow the instructions in the box. The answer to each part of the main idea question has been filled in for you. The score for each answer has also been marked.

Sample

Tangled in a wire fence, the coyote struggled to get free. Its leg was cut and bruised. The pain must have been terrible. But the animal never stopped trying to get loose.

Two young farm girls saw the trapped coyote. They hurried to a nearby house. The farmer heard their story and came to help.

They held the coyote's head in place with hoe handles. Then they cut the wire fence. The coyote slipped free. But the animal stood still. Perhaps it wanted to thank its rescuers.

The animal had to be gently nudged before it would leave. At last it hobbled off. Then it turned, pausing to look again at the good people who had saved its life.

	Answer	Score
Mark the main idea	M	10
Mark the statement that is a detail	D	5
Mark the statement that is too narrow	N	5
Mark the statement that is too broad	B	5

a. Two young girls helped to free a trapped coyote.
   [This statement is one that gathers all the important points. It gives a correct picture of the main idea in a brief way: (1) two young girls, (2) a trapped coyote, and (3) freeing it.]   M 10

b. Kind hearts set free a doomed coyote.
   [This statement is too broad. It doesn't state *who* set the coyote free. It doesn't tell *why* it was doomed.]   B 5

c. Hoe handles were used to hold the coyote's head.
   [This is just one of many details found in the passage. It has little to do with the passage as a whole.]   D 5

d. A wire fence was cut to set a coyote free.
   [Cutting the fence is *part* of the main idea. But any main idea statement must give the chief actors credit. It must mention the two girls who saved the coyote's life.]   N 5

Getting the Most Out of This Book

The following steps could be called "tricks of the trade." Your teachers might call them "rules for learning." It doesn't matter what they are called. What does matter is that they work.

Think About the Title

A famous language expert told me a "trick" to use when I read. "The first thing to do is to read the title. Then spend a few moments thinking about it."

Writers spend much time thinking up good titles. They try to pack a lot of meaning into them. It makes sense, then, for you to spend a few seconds trying to dig out some meaning. These few moments of thought will give you a head start on a passage.

Thinking about the title can help you in another way, too. It helps you concentrate on a passage before you begin reading. Why does this happen? Thinking about the title fills your head full of thoughts about the passage. There's no room for anything else to get in to break concentration.

The Dot System

Here is a method that will speed up your reading. It also builds comprehension at the same time.

Spend a few moments with the title. Then read *quickly* through the passage. Next, without looking back, answer the six questions by placing a dot in the box next to each answer of your choice. The dots will be your "unofficial" answers. For the main idea question (question six), place your dot in the box next to the statement that you think is the main idea.

The dot system helps by making you think hard on your first, *fast* reading. The practice you gain by trying to grasp and remember ideas makes you a stronger reader.

The Check-Mark System

You have now answered all of the questions with a dot. Next, read the passage once more *carefully*. This time, make your final answer to each question with a check mark (✓). Go to each question. Then, place a check mark in the box next to the answer of your choice. The answers with the check marks are the ones that will count toward your score.

Now answer the main idea question. Follow the steps that are on the question page. Use a capital letter to mark your final answer to each part of the main idea question.

The Diagnostic Chart

Now move your final answers to the Diagnostic Chart on page 102. Use the column of boxes under number *1* for the answers to the first passage. Use the column of boxes under number *2* for the answers to the second passage, and so on.

Write the letter of your answer in the *upper* part of each block.

Correct your answers using the Answer Key on pages 100 and 101. When scoring your answers, do *not* use an *x* for *incorrect* or a *c* for *correct*. Instead, use this method. If your choice is correct, make no mark in the lower part of the answer block. If your choice is *in*correct, write the letter of the correct answer in the *lower* part of the block.

Thus, the answer column for each passage will show your incorrect answers. And it will also show the correct answers.

Your Total Comprehension Score

Go back to the passage you have just read. If you answered a question incorrectly, draw a line under the correct choice on the question page. Then write your score for each question in the circle provided. Add the scores to get your Total Comprehension Score.

Graphing Your Progress

After you have found your Total Comprehension Score, turn to the Progress Graph on page 103. Write your score in the box under the number for each passage. Then put an *x* along the line above the box to show your Total Comprehension Score. Join the *x*'s as you go. This will plot a line showing your progress.

Taking Corrective Action

Your incorrect answers give you a way to teach yourself how to read better. Take the time to study your wrong answers.

Go back to the question page. Read the correct answer (the one you have underlined) several times. With the correct answer in mind, go back to the passage itself. Read to see why the approved answer is better. Try to see where you made your mistake. Try to figure out why you chose a wrong answer.

The Steps in a Nutshell

Here's a quick review of the steps to follow. Following these steps is the way to get the most out of each *Essential Skills* book. Be sure you have read and understood all of the "To the Student" section on pages 11 through 22 before you start.

1. **Think About the Title of the Passage.** Try to get all the meaning the writer put into it.
2. **Read the Passage Quickly.**
3. **Answer the Questions, Using the Dot System.** Use dots to mark your unofficial answers. Don't look back at the passage.
4. **Read the Passage Again — Carefully.**
5. **Mark Your Final Answers.** Put a check mark (✓) in the box to note your final answer. Use capital letters for each part of the main idea question.
6. **Mark Your Answers on the Diagnostic Chart.** Record your final answers in the upper blocks of the chart on page 102.
7. **Correct Your Answers.** Use the Answer Key on pages 100 and 101. If an answer is not correct, (a) write the correct answer in the lower block, beneath your wrong answer. Then (b) go back to the question page. Place a line under the correct answer.
8. **Find Your Total Comprehension Score.** Find this by adding up the points you earned for each question.
9. **Graph Your Progress.** Mark and plot your scores on the graph on page 103.
10. **Take Corrective Action.** Read your wrong answers. Read the passage once more. Try to figure out why you were wrong.

Passages and Questions

Titles of Passages

1. Vegetable Tops 24
2. From Inside the Earth 27
3. Working Together 30
4. Our Faithful Friends 33
5. Birds: Structure Means Way of Life 36
6. Woodland Detectives 39
7. The Animal With the Spiral House 42
8. The Living Turtle 45
9. Twins for Mother Moose 48
10. The Grasshopper Mouse 51
11. Christmas Trees 54
12. The Chickaree 57
13. The Sequoia Cone-Cutter 60
14. The Kingfisher 63
15. A Fish Fit for Emperors 66
16. The Eider Duck 69
17. Bats Keep Their Ears Clean 72
18. From Fawn to Yearling 75
19. Mischief-Makers 78
20. Getting Ready to Fly 81
21. The Engelmann Spruce 84
22. The Game of Sticks 87
23. Our Grasslands 90
24. The White-Footed Mouse and Its Young 93
25. Codfish 96

1. Vegetable Tops

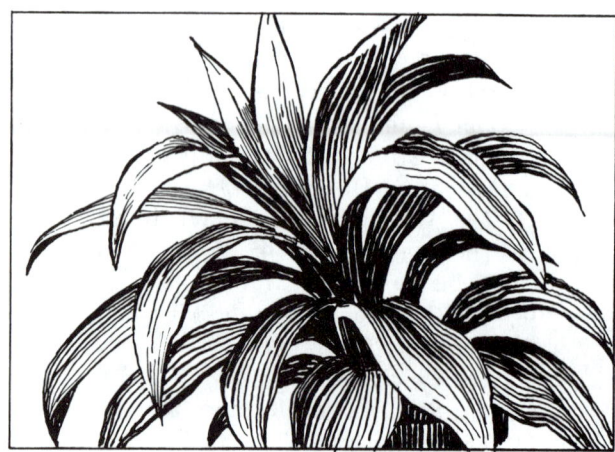

One way to grow house plants quickly and easily is to use carrot and beet tops. The leaves of the carrot plant will be light green and wispy and look like ferns. The leaves that grow from a beet top are large, dark green, and veined in deep red.

Cut a thin slice off the top of the vegetable. Remove all leaves. Place the vegetable, cut side down, in a shallow dish of water. Change the water often, and keep it about one-half inch (about 1.3 centimeters) deep. When the roots show, place the vegetable, cut side down, into a pan or pot of moist sand. Put the pot in a sunny window and watch your plant grow.

Carrot tops can also be used to make a hanging "basket". Cut off the top two inches (about 5.1 centimeters) of a large, thick carrot. Take off any leaves growing out of the top. Turn the top upside down. Push a few sewing needles with nylon thread through the side of the carrot about one-half inch (about 1.3 centimeters) down from the cut end.

Scrape out some of the carrot top's insides with a kitchen knife to make a "bowl" for holding water. Draw the threads together and knot at the top.

Fill the inside of the carrot "bowl" with water and hang in a sunny window. In a few days leaves will appear, coming from what was once the top of the carrot. Soon they will curl upward and keep growing upward around the carrot bowl. (Plants "know" which way to grow even though they're upside down!) Keep the carrot filled with water, and it will keep growing.

The hanging basket of greenery from the carrot top will become a very interesting plant. It will go well with other plants you grow from things you have saved from being thrown into garbage cans.

?

	Possible Score	Your Score

1. This passage deals mostly with

   ☐ a. pepper tops.
   ☐ b. tomato tops.
   ☐ c. carrot tops.
   ☐ d. radish tops.

   (15)

2. Beet leaves are dark green and

   ☐ a. deep red.
   ☐ b. bright yellow.
   ☐ c. purple.
   ☐ d. light orange.

   (15)

3. The leaves of the carrot and beet plants

   ☐ a. are very different.
   ☐ b. are almost the same.
   ☐ c. are exactly the same.
   ☐ d. have the same shape.

   (15)

4. A hanging basket of greenery is made of

   ☐ a. brightly colored flowers.
   ☐ b. all leaves.
   ☐ c. mostly roots.
   ☐ d. green flowers.

   (15)

5. <u>Moist</u> sand is

   ☐ a. dry.
   ☐ b. cold.
   ☐ c. wet.
   ☐ d. hot.

   (15)

6. Main Idea

	Answer	Score
Mark the main idea	M	10
Mark the statement that is a detail	D	5
Mark the statement that is too narrow	N	5
Mark the statement that is too broad	B	5

a. House plants can be grown from beet tops.

b. House plants, even hanging baskets, can be grown from carrot and beet tops.

c. New plants can be grown from pieces of the parent plant.

d. Though placed upside down, the leaves of plants will grow upward.

Total Comprehension Score
(Add your scores and enter the total on the graph on page 103.)

Categories of Comprehension Questions

No. 1: Subject Matter	No. 4: Clarifying Devices
No. 2: Supporting Details	No. 5: Vocabulary in Context
No. 3: Conclusion	No. 6: Main Idea

2. From Inside the Earth

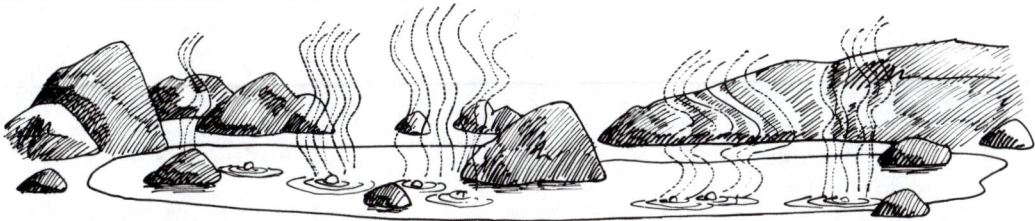

We can use the hot water and steam from inside the earth to heat our homes and to make electricity. We call this source of heat and power *geothermal* (gee oh THER mal) *energy*. We can make use of this energy when the steam or hot water comes up through cracks in the earth. We can also drill wells to tap this heat.

The people of Iceland have been using hot springs for a long time. They have built large pipes that carry the hot water to their schools and homes. Most of these schools have swimming pools heated by the springs. Some schools have heated greenhouses where plants grow. In the largest city of Iceland, nine out of ten homes get heat from this kind of energy.

On a hill in California, steam from the earth works to turn engines that make electricity for thousands of people!

We are running low on oil and gas. So the search is on for much more geothermal energy. Most of the searching is being done where there have been volcanoes and earthquakes. We know this is where the hot rock is close to the surface. There drilling won't be too deep or cost too much. Scientists are also using other ways to find hot rocks.

Even where hot rocks are found, there may be no hot water to bring up. So scientists are trying a new kind of well drilling. They drill two wells instead of one. Then they pump cold water down into the first well. The cold water flows toward the next well through cracks in the hot rocks. The water is heated by the rocks and comes up through the second well as steam or hot water.

Many people are working to find more geothermal energy because it seems to be a clean form of power. There are no strip mines to dig, no oil spills to clean up and no poisons to pile up.

But nature gives nothing for free. Using more of this type of energy will cause problems that have to be solved. For instance, there are <u>sulfides</u> and other chemicals in the steam that comes from the earth. The people who drill the wells and use the steam must take out the chemicals. This could pollute the air. One more problem is that geothermal electric plants, like all electric plants, could ruin some of our best scenery. Think of one in the middle of a place like Yellowstone Park! We must take great care when we decide where the plants can be built.

We must be careful in using geothermal energy. Still, it can help us in many ways. It may be able to give us clean power for as long as we need it. And it may help us save some oil and gas for those who will live on earth a long time from now.

_____**?**_____

	Possible Score	Your Score

1. This passage is about

   ☐ a. natural steam.
   ☐ b. strip mining.
   ☐ c. oil.
   ☐ d. natural gas.

   (15)   ○

2. For many years hot springs have been used by the people in

   ☐ a. Sweden.
   ☐ b. Russia.
   ☐ c. Greenland.
   ☐ d. Iceland.

   (15)   ○

3. If geothermal electric plants are put in the wrong place,

   ☐ a. they could run into chemical problems.
   ☐ b. they may not be pleasing to look at.
   ☐ c. they will be expensive to build.
   ☐ d. they will still add beauty to the scenery around them.

   (15)   ○

4. We are running low on oil and gas. This means that

   ☐ a. oil and gas flow like a river.
   ☐ b. the amount of oil and gas is becoming smaller.
   ☐ c. oil and gas is found deep within the earth.
   ☐ d. we need more pipes to carry oil and gas.

   (15)   ○

5. <u>Sulfides</u> are

   ☐ a. acids.
   ☐ b. vitamins.
   ☐ c. minerals.
   ☐ d. chemicals.

   (15)   ○

28

6. Main Idea

	Answer	Score
Mark the main idea	M	(10)
Mark the statement that is a detail	D	(5)
Mark the statement that is too narrow	N	(5)
Mark the statement that is too broad	B	(5)

a. In California, steam from within the earth is used to turn engines to make electricity.

b. Some form of energy is needed to replace the oil and gas we are using up.

c. Steam, hot water, or hot rocks from within the earth can provide us with a new form of energy.

d. Chemicals such as sulfides are found in the steam from within the earth.

Total Comprehension Score
(Add your scores and enter the total on the graph on page 103.)

Categories of Comprehension Questions

No. 1: Subject Matter	No. 4: Clarifying Devices
No. 2: Supporting Details	No. 5: Vocabulary in Context
No. 3: Conclusion	No. 6: Main Idea

29

3. Working Together

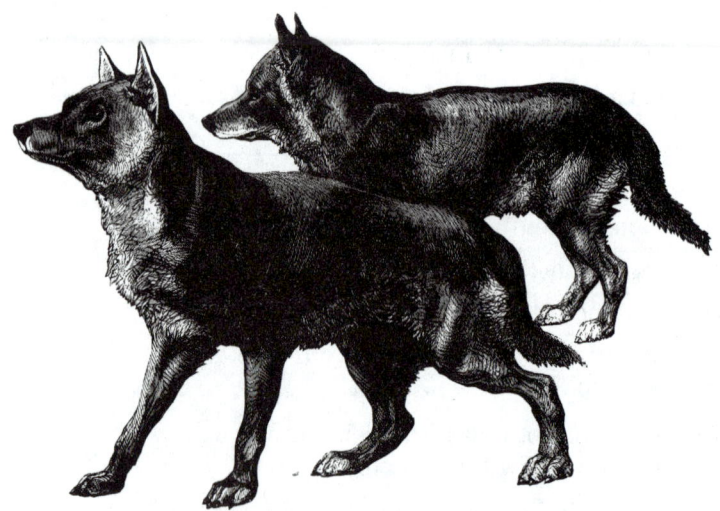

Life in the wild dog pack is very peaceful. There is no fighting between the dogs, no matter how many share the kill. Sometimes a lame or sick dog arrives too late for the meal. It must beg for food from one or more pack members. Some of the dogs will then share the meat they have already eaten by throwing up some of it for their hungry friend.

Once a year a female in the pack has pups. There may be as many as sixteen in a litter. The pack finds a den — often an empty hyena burrow — in which the pups are born. Here they stay until the pups are three to four months old and are able to travel with the pack. The pack usually goes hunting at dawn or sometimes in the late evening. During this time, several dogs stay behind and guard the pups. This dividing of the work is unusual in mammals.

Wild dogs are good hunters. They usually do not return without having killed. When they return to the den, they feed not only the pups but also the guards by throwing up chunks of meat carried home in their stomachs.

When the pups are old enough to travel, they trail behind the hunting pack. After a kill has been made, they run up and take over the whole carcass. They eat until they are full while the adults wait for any scraps that may be left. Often, nothing is left when the pups are done, and the pack must hunt again.

_____ **?** _____

	Possible Score / Your Score

1. This passage talks about the wild dog as

    ☐ a. a selfish animal.
    ☑ b. a parent and hunter.
    ☐ c. a species that is dying out.
    ☐ d. an enemy of humans.

    (15)   ◯

2. Female dogs often give birth in

    ☑ a. empty hyena burrows.
    ☐ b. small underground caves.
    ☐ c. thick bushes.
    ☐ d. hollow tree trunks.

    (15)   ◯

3. The wild dog seems to be

    ☐ a. full of revenge and anger.
    ☐ b. uninterested in caring for its family.
    ☐ c. mean and ill-tempered.
    ☑ d. a loyal member of the pack.

    (15)   ◯

4. The last paragraph describes the pack's

    ☐ a. mating habits.
    ☐ b. size.
    ☑ c. eating habits.
    ☐ d. leader.

    (15)   ◯

5. As used in this passage, a <u>carcass</u> is

    ☑ a. the body of a dead animal.
    ☐ b. a wounded dog.
    ☐ c. a young dog.
    ☐ d. the entire wild dog pack.

    (15)   ◯

6. Main Idea

	Answer	Score
Mark the main idea	M	10
Mark the statement that is a detail	D	5
Mark the statement that is too narrow	N	5
Mark the statement that is too broad	B	5

a. The pack usually hunts at dawn or late evening.

b. Some dogs will share their meal with a lame friend.

c. Wild dogs do not fight one another.

d. Members of a wild dog pack take good care of each other.

Total Comprehension Score
(Add your scores and enter the total on the graph on page 103.)

Categories of Comprehension Questions

No. 1: Subject Matter	No. 4: Clarifying Devices
No. 2: Supporting Details	No. 5: Vocabulary in Context
No. 3: Conclusion	No. 6: Main Idea

4. Our Faithful Friends

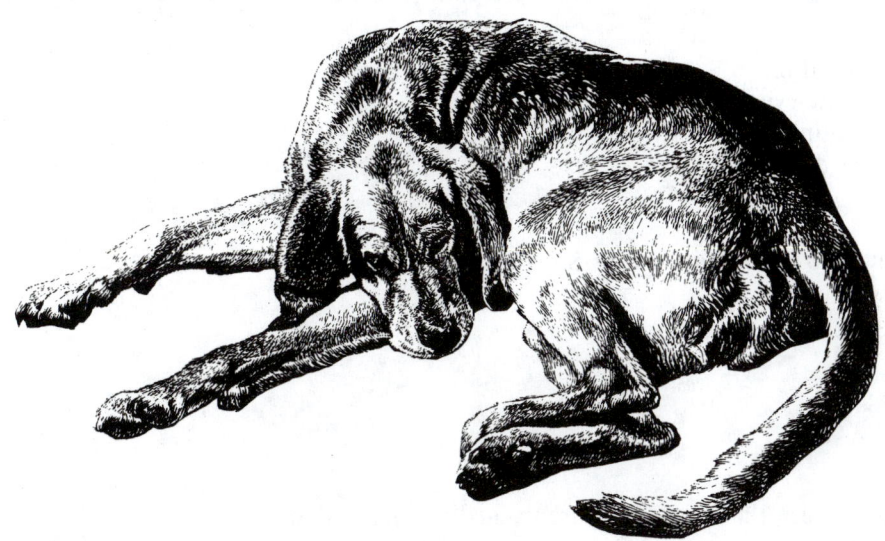

People have had tame dogs for a long, long time. No one knows just where they were first tamed or who first tamed them. Many scientists say that tame dogs come from the Eurasian wolves of long ago and from the jackals of Africa and southern Asia.

Some of the dogs changed in form after people tamed them. Then people chose certain kinds of dogs to mate with other kinds. Today, we have around 200 species or types of dogs.

Our pet dogs inherited fine traits from their ancestors and closest relatives, the wolves. They love to run and hunt and are skillful fighters. They are brave in protecting those they love, and they show great affection.

Most domestic dogs are smart. They can be trained to do many things. Besides being used for hunting, they can be taught to be watchdogs or guides for blind people. In some countries they are used to herd livestock. In other places, they pull sleds through snow or help hunt for lost people.

Besides their other skills, dogs can talk to each other. Wild dogs greet a visiting dog with friendly tail-waving and happy sounds of welcome. But they drive away a threatening animal with leaps and growls.

Your dog "talks" to other dogs and to you when it sniffs, whines, growls, barks or wags its tail. As you get to know your dog, you will learn when it is hungry or wants to be let out or in. You will be able to tell if it is hurt or unhappy and when it wants to play. The more you try to understand your dog, the more it will repay you with affection.

_____ **?** _____

	Possible Score	Your Score

1. The subject of this passage is

    ☐ a. wild dogs.
    ☐ b. seeing-eye dogs.
    ☐ c. hunting dogs.
    ☐ d. pet dogs.

    15

2. About how many types of dogs do we have today?

    ☐ a. 100
    ☐ b. 150
    ☐ c. 200
    ☐ d. 300

    15

3. It can be seen that tame dogs are trained for many things because

    ☐ a. of their size.
    ☐ b. they are smart.
    ☐ c. they can communicate.
    ☐ d. of their friendly character.

    15

4. Wolves are "skillful fighters" which means

    ☐ a. they do not fight.
    ☐ b. they are good at fighting.
    ☐ c. they will run away from a fight.
    ☐ d. they are shy.

    15

5. A good synonym for <u>domestic</u> is

    ☐ a. wild.
    ☐ b. hunting.
    ☐ c. tame.
    ☐ d. powerful.

    15

6. Main Idea

	Answer	Score
Mark the main idea	M	(10)
Mark the statement that is a detail	D	(5)
Mark the statement that is too narrow	N	(5)
Mark the statement that is too broad	B	(5)

a. Dogs have many skills which are useful to people including the ability to communicate.

b. There are about 200 species or types of dogs.

c. Dogs are very skillful animals.

d. Dogs tell a visiting dog that it is welcome with tail-wagging and happy sounds.

Total Comprehension Score
(Add your scores and enter the total on the graph on page 103.)

Categories of Comprehension Questions

No. 1: Subject Matter	No. 4: Clarifying Devices
No. 2: Supporting Details	No. 5: Vocabulary in Context
No. 3: Conclusion	No. 6: Main Idea

5. Birds: Structure Means Way of Life

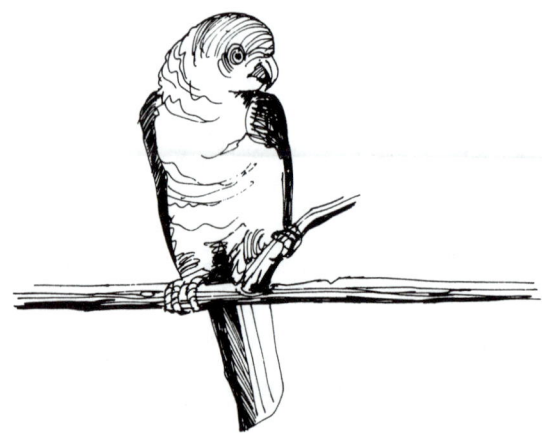

A bird's structure suits it to a certain way of life. For example, all birds are able to perch in some fashion. But you never see a hawk perched on a telephone wire. This is because its foot and leg structure are better for food-getting than for perching. Thus, hawks use their feet to catch and carry food, not to perch.

Some birds developed feet with long, strong toes that could grasp rough bark to help them climb straight up a tree. Some of these also had hard bills to peck into wood and reach insects. These birds are woodpeckers. They are built for pecking at trees. And that is how they live.

Predatory birds, such as hawks, are excellent fliers with powerful legs and feet. So they can fly for hours or even days searching for food; and when they see a rodent or rabbit, they can pin it down with razor-sharp talons. The duck hawk is built strong and fast. So it is able to kill its prey in midair with one punch of its feet. Then it can catch it before it reaches the ground! Strong, hooked bills suit hawks and owls to tear apart large prey which they can't swallow whole. So they like to hunt large prey.

Birds have exceptionally good vision. This suits them to certain eating habits. A sharp-eyed chimney swift can catch tiny insects as it flies. Red-tailed hawks can detect field mice a quarter of a mile away. Thus, mice are its main food. Great horned owls can see ten times better than we can in dim light. So they are night hunters. Birds' eyes are enormous for the small size of their skulls. If their skulls were as large as ours, their eyes would be as big as tennis balls. Owls and other night-flying species possess the largest eyes, while birds we see in our gardens possess the smallest.

A bird's hearing also influences its eating habits. Owls have the best hearing. So in total darkness they can fly directly to a mouse as it makes a light rustle among the dry leaves.

It is easy to see that different structures can mean different ways of living. And it is interesting to find that each bird has its own way of life.

_____ ? _____

	Possible Score	Your Score

1. This passage is about

   ☐ a. the naming of birds.
   ☐ b. birds' structures and habits.
   ☐ c. the ways birds build nests.
   ☐ d. how birds are banded.

   (15)   ◯

2. A hawk often feeds on

   ☐ a. fish.
   ☐ b. small animals.
   ☐ c. insects.
   ☐ d. other birds.

   (15)   ◯

3. Predatory birds seem to eat mostly

   ☐ a. seeds.
   ☐ b. insects.
   ☐ c. plants.
   ☐ d. meat.

   (15)   ◯

4. The writer mentions the great horned owl to show

   ☐ a. that birds have good vision.
   ☐ b. how birds hunt.
   ☐ c. where a bird's ears are located.
   ☐ d. how some birds carry food.

   (15)   ◯

5. <u>Talons</u> refer to a bird's

   ☐ a. bill.
   ☐ b. legs.
   ☐ c. eyes.
   ☐ d. claws.

   (15)   ◯

37

6. Main Idea

	Answer	Score
Mark the main idea	M	10
Mark the statement that is a detail	D	5
Mark the statement that is too narrow	N	5
Mark the statement that is too broad	B	5

a. The red-tailed hawk can see a mouse a quarter of a mile (about .4 kilometers) away; thus, it feeds on mice.

b. The way a bird is built suits it to a certain kind of life.

c. All birds are designed to survive in the wild.

d. A duck hawk is able to kill its prey in midair and catch it before it reaches the ground.

Total Comprehension Score
(Add your scores and enter the total on the graph on page 103.)

Categories of Comprehension Questions

No. 1: Subject Matter	No. 4: Clarifying Devices
No. 2: Supporting Details	No. 5: Vocabulary in Context
No. 3: Conclusion	No. 6: Main Idea

6. Woodland Detectives

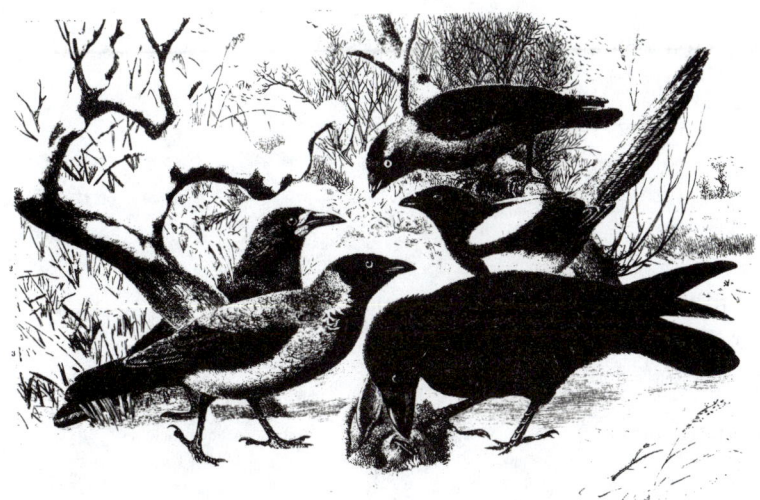

Now that winter is here, don't crawl into a hole and hibernate as some animals do. Bundle up in your warmest clothes and go out into the woods. A walk in the winter woods can be fun.

Did you ever look closely at chewed branches of shrubs and trees? The special toothmarks that animals leave give them away. A bunny makes a clean cut while a deer tears a twig. The deer's upper teeth are not good for cutting.

Under a large pine tree you may see big chips of wood lying on the snow. This is your signal to look up the trunk. You may see the holes made by a woodpecker. When one of these birds goes after food (an insect??) buried in the trunk, it hammers out those wood chips with its strong beak.

Over in the bushes is a huge ice cream cone! A bird's nest, left from last summer, caught the soft snow and held it — white against the black twigs. When we brush off the snow to peek, it looks like someone's leftover lunch inside. A mouse has moved in for the winter.

Farther along where some fruits have fallen from the berry bushes, the mice have paid a visit. Their dizzy tracks go in and out over the snow and finally end at a hole. The heat of their little bodies has frosted the edge, trimming it in icy lace.

Chickadees hop from branch to branch among the birches, knocking down a shower of seeds. As if by magic, the tiny seeds on the snow look like a skyful of airplanes.

If it is late winter and you think spring is never going to come, just look up around you at the tips of branches. You will be surprised to see so much color. The red maple buds look almost ready to burst, and soon the sap will be rising in the sugar maples.

_____ **?** _____

		Possible Score	Your Score

1. This passage talks about the woods in

    ☐ a. summer.
    ☐ b. fall.
    ☐ c. winter.
    ☐ d. spring.   15   ◯

2. According to this passage you can tell one animal from another by its

    ☐ a. fur.
    ☐ b. toothmarks.
    ☐ c. tracks.
    ☐ d. call.   15   ◯

3. We can see from the last paragraph that

    ☐ a. many trees die in winter.
    ☐ b. sugar maples are tall trees.
    ☐ c. trees tell the coming of spring.
    ☐ d. red maples grow anywhere.   15   ◯

4. The "ice cream cone" in this passage is a

    ☐ a. large, white rock.
    ☐ b. bright pink sunset.
    ☐ c. snow-covered nest.
    ☐ d. white rabbit on a stump.   15   ◯

5. Another word for <u>huge</u> is

    ☐ a. cold.
    ☐ b. large.
    ☐ c. soft.
    ☐ d. tiny.   15   ◯

6. Main Idea

	Answer	Score
Mark the main idea	M	10
Mark the statement that is a detail	D	5
Mark the statement that is too narrow	N	5
Mark the statement that is too broad	B	5

a. A winter walk through the woods reveals evidence of the creatures which live there.

b. A walk can lead to the discovery of many things.

c. Chips of wood show where a woodpecker looked for food buried in a tree trunk.

d. Tiny seeds on the snow look like airplanes in the sky.

Total Comprehension Score
(Add your scores and enter the total on the graph on page 103.)

Categories of Comprehension Questions

No. 1: Subject Matter	No. 4: Clarifying Devices
No. 2: Supporting Details	No. 5: Vocabulary in Context
No. 3: Conclusion	No. 6: Main Idea

7. The Animal With the Spiral House

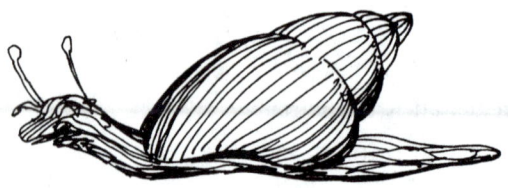

What animal walks on one foot, has a mouth like a file, a body twisted like a screw and, though it never makes a sound, always leaves a trail? A snail!

There are both land and water snails. Land snails have lungs and breathe air. Most water snails have gills, somewhat like those of a fish, which get oxygen from the water. Some water snails have lungs and must come to the surface to breathe air through a tube that serves as a built-in snorkel. Many can even leave the water and move about on land.

Land snails are common in the woods. However, you won't find them in evergreen forests because the soil is too acidic. Most stay hidden in the soil or under fallen trees or decaying leaves. They are often the same color as the soil or leaves.

Because their bodies must be kept moist, snails usually stay in the shade, but on cloudy, damp days, you may find one searching for food in the open.

Water snails can be found clinging to plants and rocks in almost any body of water. Since the water prevents them from drying out, they can be found moving about all through the day.

Don't be afraid to pick up a snail — it can't bite. While you're holding the snail, look at its shell. The snail carries its home around on its back and can pull back into its shell for protection against many enemies. Also, when its surroundings get cold or dry, it can pull inside and sleep.

Its shell always grows in a spiral. It grows around and around, getting bigger as it turns. As the animal grows, it makes a larger shell.

When the snail pokes out of its shell, look at it. It won't be afraid of you, because it doesn't really "see" as you do. Most snails can see only if there is a change in the light.

On the bottom of the snail's body is its mouth. It has a file-like tongue called a *radula* (RAJ oo luh) which is covered with many tiny teeth. It uses this radula to scrape small bits of food into its mouth.

Another part on the bottom of its body is its traveling pad, called its *foot*. Set the snail down on something and it seems to just flow along like a snake. It doesn't have any legs and doesn't need any. Put it on a pane of glass and watch it from the other side. You will soon see muscular waves pass down its foot, carrying the snail forward. It helps itself by secreting slime which makes it easier to slide along.

?

	Possible Score	Your Score

1. What would be another good title for this passage?

    ☐ a. Facts about Snails
    ☐ b. Snails and Shellfish
    ☐ c. The Damaging Snail
    ☐ d. The Snail — A Special Treat

    (15)　○

2. Snails must keep their bodies

    ☐ a. clean.
    ☐ b. dry.
    ☐ c. moist.
    ☐ d. oiled.

    (15)　○

3. Snails are

    ☐ a. harmless.
    ☐ b. curious.
    ☐ c. tricky.
    ☐ d. noisy.

    (15)　○

4. A "spiral shell" is shaped like

    ☐ a. a saw.
    ☐ b. a wrench.
    ☐ c. a screw.
    ☐ d. a hammer.

    (15)　○

5. Decaying leaves are

    ☐ a. interesting leaves.
    ☐ b. moving leaves.
    ☐ c. budding leaves.
    ☐ d. rotting leaves.

    (15)　○

6. Main Idea

	Answer	Score
Mark the main idea	M	10
Mark the statement that is a detail	D	5
Mark the statement that is too narrow	N	5
Mark the statement that is too broad	B	5

a. Land snails are often the same color as the soil or leaves.

b. Some creatures can live both in water and on land.

c. Snails are interesting creatures which are found in water and on land.

d. Snails move in an unusual way.

Total Comprehension Score
(Add your scores and enter the total on the graph on page 103.)

Categories of Comprehension Questions

No. 1: Subject Matter	No. 4: Clarifying Devices
No. 2: Supporting Details	No. 5: Vocabulary in Context
No. 3: Conclusion	No. 6: Main Idea

8. The Living Turtle

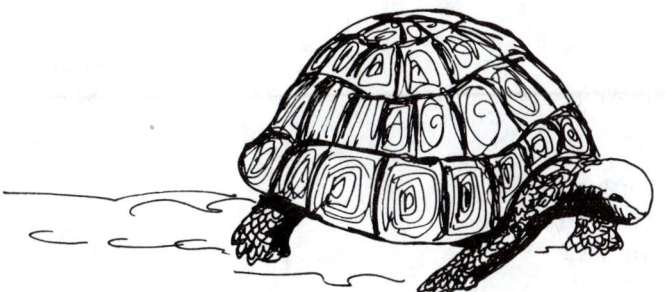

How and what do turtles eat? Turtles don't move fast enough to chase anything, and they have no teeth. They have a hard bony edge where the teeth should be. The edge may be smooth or rough. In some turtles, such as the box turtle, the upper lip is shaped like a stubby beak. Their jaw muscles are so strong that even without teeth they can cut, tear, crunch or mash many things. Most will eat insects if one is careless enough to sit while the turtle makes a slow grab. Worms, grubs, small fish, crabs and a variety of plant life, including berries and fruit, are also food for turtles.

Some turtles are *herbivores* (plant eaters), whereas others are *omnivores* (plant and meat eaters). The snapping turtle, for example, often watches for a chance to sneak up under an unsuspecting duckling, grab its leg and pull the bird underwater for a meal.

How are turtles born? All turtles are hatched from eggs. The female digs a hole in the ground. The land turtle lays six to twelve, nearly round, leathery-shelled eggs. Turtles that live in the ocean lay many more eggs but come ashore to lay them. Once the eggs are laid, the female covers them with soil or sand and leaves. She never bothers with them again.

Turtle eggs are good to eat, and many predators sniff them out, dig them up and have a feast. People often hunt for sea turtle nests and steal the eggs. The eggs that survive are incubated by the warmth of the sun on the ground. In about two months they hatch. The little ones scramble out ready to take care of themselves at once. If they are aquatic turtles, they head for the nearest water. If they are land turtles, they find a hiding place for a short time while their little shells harden, and they examine their new world.

Where do turtles live? Depending on the kind, turtles live in temperate or tropic areas. Some, such as the wood turtle, like damp, shady woodlands. Others prefer sunny meadows. A quiet pond or stream edge may have several kinds of turtles. Turtles can be found in the oceans and along seashores, in desert areas and quite often in your own back yard, garden or nearby park.

Some spend most or all of their time in the water. Others spend more time on land. Most seem to enjoy basking in the sun. Even those who live in the water come out on the shore from time to time to sunbathe or to lay eggs.

Turtles mature in five to seven years. Unless they meet a predator, a car or a thoughtless human, they have an average life-span of forty to fifty years. However, there are records of turtles in captivity that have lived up to 150 years.

?

	Possible Score	Your Score

1. This passage deals with

   ☐ a. turtle grass.
   ☐ b. the uses of turtle meat.
   ☐ c. the sea tortoise and its shell.
   ☐ d. facts about turtles.

   15

2. According to this passage, all turtles

   ☐ a. are meat eaters.
   ☐ b. hibernate.
   ☐ c. hatch from eggs.
   ☐ d. live in the water.

   15

3. Young turtles

   ☐ a. are not cared for by either parent.
   ☐ b. are often eaten by their parents.
   ☐ c. need much care and are very helpless.
   ☐ d. are fully grown the day they are born.

   15

4. The second sentence tell us that turtles

   ☐ a. are very slow creatures.
   ☐ b. have sharp teeth.
   ☐ c. chase their food.
   ☐ d. don't eat much.

   15

5. <u>Aquatic</u> turtles live

   ☐ a. on the desert.
   ☐ b. in the woods.
   ☐ c. in a zoo.
   ☐ d. in or near water.

   15

6. Main Idea

	Answer	Score
Mark the main idea	M	10
Mark the statement that is a detail	D	5
Mark the statement that is too narrow	N	5
Mark the statement that is too broad	B	5

a. A single species can contain great variety among the creatures in its group.

b. Turtles are interesting animals with a variety of living habits.

c. If not eaten, turtle eggs hatch in about 2 months.

d. Some turtles are plant eaters; some are plant and meat eaters.

Total Comprehension Score
(Add your scores and enter the total on the graph on page 103.)

Categories of Comprehension Questions

No. 1: Subject Matter	No. 4: Clarifying Devices
No. 2: Supporting Details	No. 5: Vocabulary in Context
No. 3: Conclusion	No. 6: Main Idea

47

9. Twins for Mother Moose

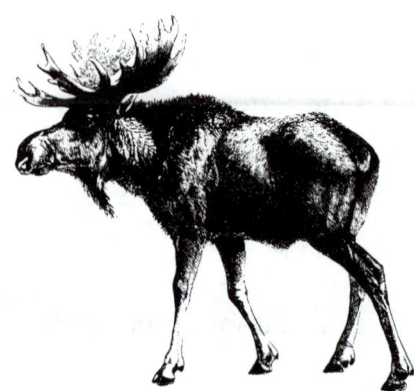

Alces (AL cease) the moose had twin calves in late May. All around her the trees and bushes of eastern Canada sparkled with new, lime-green leaves. Fresh watercress floated in the nearby streams. This summer would be rich with food for the moose.

The calves' father fed on willow leaves. He was a huge bull moose who weighed more than 1,500 pounds (about 680.4 kilograms) and stood about six and a half feet (about 2 meters) tall at the shoulders. During the fall he had had huge antlers that looked like strange, outstretched hands. He had shed them in the winter, and now a new set was growing. They were covered with *velvet,* a thin skin which supplied the growing antlers with the blood they needed.

Normally, the bull moose lived by himself in the river valleys and swamps, but he had stayed with Alces since they mated in early autumn. Now that the calves were born, he would go his own way.

Alces proved to be a good mother. For the calves' first two weeks she kept them hidden in bushes along one of the streams. Like baby deer, they had no telltale odor that might attract enemies, but Alces stayed close to them anyway. She spent much of her time belly-deep in the stream, dipping her huge head under the surface. She pulled at the sweet, fresh watercress and pondweed; or she wandered among the willows, munching on the new shoots.

When the twins were two weeks old, they left their hiding place and followed Alces as she worked her way through the wet bottomlands of the stream.

Alces looked much the same as other moose, the largest members of the deer family. She had a huge muzzle, as do all moose, which overhung her upper lip. A flap of skin called a *bell* hung from her neck. She was dark brown with slightly lighter undersides. She had long legs and broad hoofs.

_____ **?** _____

	Possible Score	Your Score

1. This passage talks mainly about

   ☐ a. the male moose.
   ☐ b. the moose herd.
   ☐ c. the female moose.
   ☐ d. moose and deer.

   (15) ◯

2. Moose mate in the

   ☐ a. summer.
   ☐ b. autumn.
   ☐ c. winter.
   ☐ d. spring.

   (15) ◯

3. Watercress grows

   ☐ a. under rocks.
   ☐ b. on the ocean floor.
   ☐ c. in open fields.
   ☐ d. in fresh water.

   (15) ◯

4. The mother moose was munching on some "new shoots." In this passage "new shoots" are

   ☐ a. hunters.
   ☐ b. baby moose.
   ☐ c. antlers.
   ☐ d. young plants.

   (15) ◯

5. A <u>bull</u> moose is a

   ☐ a. male moose.
   ☐ b. sick moose.
   ☐ c. baby moose.
   ☐ d. runaway moose.

   (15) ◯

6. Main Idea

	Answer	Score
Mark the main idea	M	10
Mark the statement that is a detail	D	5
Mark the statement that is too narrow	N	5
Mark the statement that is too broad	B	5

a. Alces proved to be a good mother.

b. Most mothers care for their young.

c. Alces stayed close to her twin calves.

d. Baby calves of moose have no telltale odor.

Total Comprehension Score
(Add your scores and enter the
total on the graph on page 103.)

Categories of Comprehension Questions

No. 1: Subject Matter	No. 4: Clarifying Devices
No. 2: Supporting Details	No. 5: Vocabulary in Context
No. 3: Conclusion	No. 6: Main Idea

10. The Grasshopper Mouse

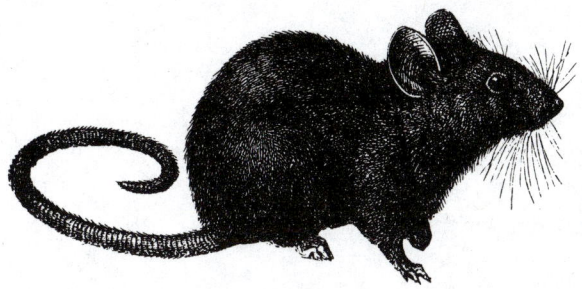

The grasshopper mouse likes to eat other kinds of mice. This mouse has a chunky body not built for speed. Other mice can most often outrun it. But the grasshopper mouse makes a quick meal of any mouse it can corner or sneak up to and pounce on.

The grasshopper mouse is a pinkish brown color, with a pure white belly and a white-tipped tail. It makes its home in the deserts and plains of the North American West. It is well suited to life where there is little rain. This mouse gets much of the water it needs from the bodies of the animals it eats. It seldom needs to take a drink.

In one night a grasshopper mouse will eat nearly its own weight in food if it has the chance. The little creature has no trouble digesting the tough, shell-like hides of many beetles and other insects. This hunter likes to kill its own prey rather than feed on animals that are already dead.

While most mice are seen as foes by humans, grasshopper mice are welcomed by many people. The wise farmer knows that this squat little mouse is a friend. It will eat many insect pests and mice which harm crops.

With its strong, sharp front claws the grasshopper mouse can dig a burrow. And it often does. But it also may use the empty homes of prairie dogs, kangaroo rats and other animals that nest below ground to escape the hot sun.

In the spring or early summer, the female lines a snug burrow with soft grass or shredded leaves. There she will give birth to about three tiny mice. The babies are naked and helpless at birth. Each is about the size of a pea. They grow quickly, though. In less than a month, they are on their own.

Young grasshopper mice and their parents, too, need sensitive noses and keen hearing. Owls, coyotes, bobcats and other nighttime hunters love to eat mouse meat for dinner!

_____ **?** _____

	Possible Score	Your Score

1. This passage is mostly about the grasshopper mouse and its

   ☐ a. young.
   ☐ b. eating habits.
   ☐ c. cousin, the field mouse.
   ☐ d. enemies.

   15   ◯

2. Where does the grasshopper mouse live?

   ☐ a. Near the coast
   ☐ b. In mountainous areas
   ☐ c. Around swampy regions
   ☐ d. In deserts and plains

   15   ◯

3. After reading this passage, we can guess that this mouse

   ☐ a. has a big appetite.
   ☐ b. can outrun most mice.
   ☐ c. eats a lot of corn.
   ☐ d. lives in trees.

   15   ◯

4. Which of the following shows how the wise farmer feels toward the grasshopper mouse?

   ☐ a. Dislike
   ☐ b. Grateful
   ☐ c. Unconcerned
   ☐ d. Angry

   15   ◯

5. As used in this passage, squat means

   ☐ a. tall and heavy.
   ☐ b. dark.
   ☐ c. cinnamon color.
   ☐ d. short and fat.

   15   ◯

6. Main Idea

	Answer	Score
Mark the main idea	M	10
Mark the statement that is a detail	D	5
Mark the statement that is too narrow	N	5
Mark the statement that is too broad	B	5

a. A grasshopper mouse will eat nearly its own weight in insects and mice.

b. Some mice are not considered enemies or pests by human beings.

c. At birth, baby grasshopper mice are about the size of a pea.

d. The grasshopper mouse is an interesting creature which helps farmers by eating mice and insects.

Total Comprehension Score
(Add your scores and enter the total on the graph on page 103.)

Categories of Comprehension Questions

No. 1: Subject Matter	No. 4: Clarifying Devices
No. 2: Supporting Details	No. 5: Vocabulary in Context
No. 3: Conclusion	No. 6: Main Idea

11. Christmas Trees

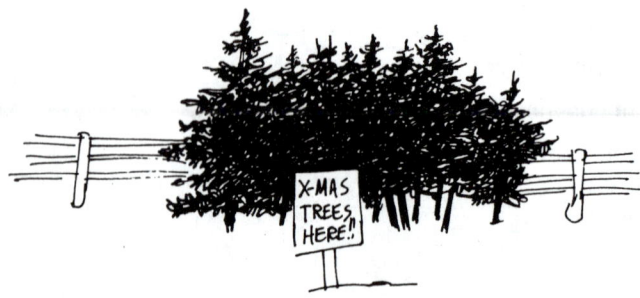

Buying live Christmas trees is a great idea. But for people who have no place to plant them, cut Christmas trees are just fine. Using them doesn't really hurt our forests. You see, most Christmas trees are grown in special places called *Christmas tree farms*.

The trees on these farms are planted, nourished, pruned and cut just for Christmas. The trees from such farms are four to six feet (about 1.2 to 1.8 meters) tall and are close to ten years old. They have been well taken care of; they are full and well shaped. And they can hold all your ornaments!

Most people think a Christmas tree is a Christmas tree — and that's all there is to it. But do you know that six different kinds of evergreens are used for Christmas trees? Not all are grown on farms. Some come from forests that have been thinned out to make more growing room for the trees which are left.

The Scotch pine was brought from Europe long ago. It grows quickly in dry, infertile soil. It has become a beautiful, bushy tree by the time it reaches your house.

The red pine is known by its reddish brown bark. It grows straight and fast on many Christmas tree farms in the northern part of the country.

The Douglas fir grows in the western part of the country on both sides of the Rockies. Douglas firs can grow to be about 300 feet (about 91 meters) tall.

Black spruce makes a fine, small, table tree. These trees grow slowly in the bogs of the north. Besides the trees being used at Christmas, their sticky "resin" is used in making chewing gum and their wood in making paper.

The balsam fir is quite popular because its spicy odor brings the woods right indoors. Also, its needles stay on the tree for a long time after the presents are all unwrapped.

Eastern red cedars are really junipers that can grow about 100 feet (about 30.5 meters) tall. If the soil is poor, though, the trees grow only to the size of a bush. The blue-gray berries have a clean, spicy smell if you crush them between your fingers.

No matter what part of the country your tree comes from, it was probably grown just for Christmas.

?

			Possible Score	Your Score

1. What would be another good title for this passage?

    ☐ a. Kinds of Christmas Trees
    ☐ b. How Much Is That Tree?
    ☐ c. Plastics Made from Trees
    ☐ d. Evergreens Never Die

    (15)

2. A Christmas tree which is 4–6 feet (about 1.2–1.8 meters) tall is close to

    ☐ a. 2 years old.
    ☐ b. 5 years old.
    ☐ c. 8 years old.
    ☐ d. 10 years old.

    (15)

3. Because of Christmas tree farms,

    ☐ a. evergreens will probably never become extinct.
    ☐ b. more and more artificial trees are being bought.
    ☐ c. the price of Christmas trees has come down.
    ☐ d. many people refuse to buy real trees.

    (15)

4. The second paragraph tells us about

    ☐ a. Christmas tree farms.
    ☐ b. Scotch pines.
    ☐ c. artificial trees.
    ☐ d. tree ornaments.

    (15)

5. A <u>bushy</u> tree is

    ☐ a. sickly.
    ☐ b. small and thin.
    ☐ c. full and thick.
    ☐ d. very short.

    (15)

6. Main Idea

	Answer	Score
Mark the main idea	M	10
Mark the statement that is a detail	D	5
Mark the statement that is too narrow	N	5
Mark the statement that is too broad	B	5

a. Douglas firs can grow to be about 300 feet (about 91 meters) tall.

b. The red pine tree grows on Christmas tree farms in the northern United States.

c. Of the 6 kinds of trees used for Christmas trees, most are grown on special farms.

d. Some trees are grown for special purposes.

Total Comprehension Score
(Add your scores and enter the total on the graph on page 103.)

Categories of Comprehension Questions

No. 1: Subject Matter	No. 4: Clarifying Devices
No. 2: Supporting Details	No. 5: Vocabulary in Context
No. 3: Conclusion	No. 6: Main Idea

12. The Chickaree

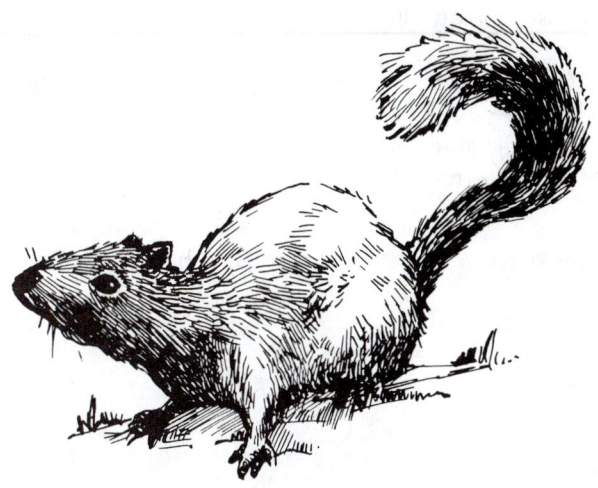

The male chickaree squirrel seems to know each knothole, twig, rock, bush and clump of grass in his territory. He will not step into another squirrel's land unless he is chasing off an <u>intruder</u>. If he does, he will be chased by the squirrel that lives there.

The chickaree is named after the sound that he makes. He spends most of his life in the trees. A black line divides his gray coat and brown belly. But he looks just like a gray blur as he runs along the branches and up the trunk. To come down a tree, he trots with his forelegs while his hindlegs act as brakes. He can jump eight feet to another branch by spreading his tail and legs flat out. If he falls, he twists like a cat until he's right side up. Landing on his feet, he's up and away in a flash.

Smallest of the tree squirrels, the chickaree builds one or more huge leafy nests in the fork of a tree branch. Then he weaves needles, moss, leaves and twigs into a rounded windproof and rainproof home as large as a bread box. His living room, lined inside with soft shredded bark, is smaller than a loaf of bread. He "closes" his door with a curtain of moss.

Though he grooms himself often, he is bothered by fleas and mites. He has to move to another nest from time to time to starve out the pests.

In early spring he looks around to find a mate. Instead of screaming insults, he calls softly. A female will let him enter her territory for that day *only*.

After they have mated, the female might move to an empty woodpecker's hole. Here, from four to seven babies are born. The mother then moves them to a leafy nest near the edge of her territory. The young squirrels stay with her for the summer. By fall they are looking for their own territories.

?

	Possible Score	Your Score

1. This passage discusses mostly the

   ☐ a. enemies of the chickaree.
   ☐ b. chickaree's nest.
   ☐ c. eating habits of the squirrel.
   ☐ d. prey of the tree squirrel.

   15

2. A squirrel may move from his nest because he is bothered by

   ☐ a. other squirrels.
   ☐ b. falling leaves.
   ☐ c. fleas and mites.
   ☐ d. birds.

   15

3. This passage suggests that squirrels live alone except for

   ☐ a. hunting.
   ☐ b. one day of mating.
   ☐ c. feeding.
   ☐ d. gathering acorns.

   15

4. The chickaree looks like a blur as he gallops along branches. This means

   ☐ a. he stops often.
   ☐ b. he is slow.
   ☐ c. he moves very fast.
   ☐ d. he walks carefully.

   15

5. An <u>intruder</u> is someone who

   ☐ a. is lazy.
   ☐ b. enters another's territory.
   ☐ c. is frightened.
   ☐ d. hunts.

   15

6. Main Idea

	Answer	Score
Mark the main idea	M	10
Mark the statement that is a detail	D	5
Mark the statement that is too narrow	N	5
Mark the statement that is too broad	B	5

a. There are many interesting creatures found in nature.

b. A chickaree has a gray coat with a brown belly.

c. A chickaree is a squirrel with interesting living habits.

d. The chickaree keeps strictly to his own territory except to mate.

Total Comprehension Score
(Add your scores and enter the total on the graph on page 103.)

Categories of Comprehension Questions

No. 1: Subject Matter	No. 4: Clarifying Devices
No. 2: Supporting Details	No. 5: Vocabulary in Context
No. 3: Conclusion	No. 6: Main Idea

13. The Sequoia Cone-Cutter

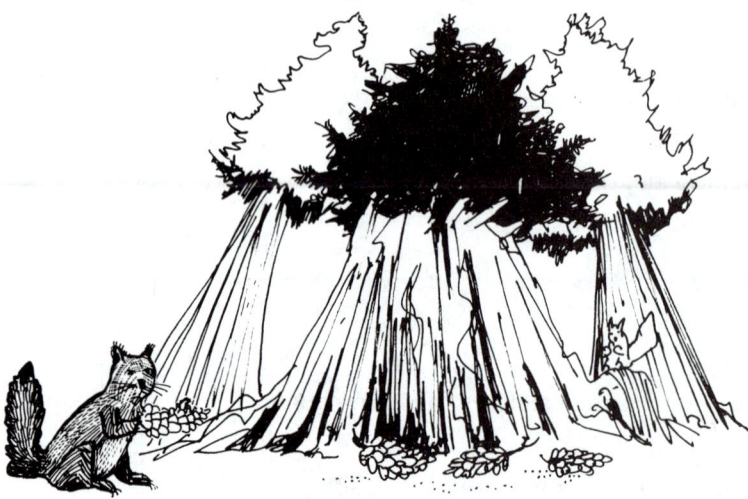

It looks as if there's a mad squirrel loose. You can see it in California in a forest on the western slopes of the Sierra Nevada mountains. It runs up a sequoia tree . . . up, up, up as high as twenty houses stacked on top of each other. It cuts off a tender green cone and bites into it like a small jackhammer. Seeds and pieces of cone fall to the ground.

It cuts these cones for winter storage. They fall to the earth like hail the size of lemons. In the time it takes you to watch a movie, it can cut enough cones to fill your bathtub. While you eat lunch, it can fill your wastebasket.

This scamp of the Sierra is the chickaree, or Douglas squirrel. And it does more than it knows. It's keeping alive the great species of giant sequoia, the largest of all living things!

This tree is so huge that if it were to grow on your own lawn, the trunk might cover your whole yard. It could be more than thirty feet (about 9.1 meters) thick. Yet its seeds are so small that it takes 1,200 of them to fill a teaspoon.

The chickaree eats the outer part of the sequoia cone itself and leaves the tiny seeds. Due to its sloppy table manners, it spills the seeds on the ground. Seeds fall from dry cones, too, but they aren't as fertile. That means that the seeds which the chickaree separates from the cones are more likely to sprout and start a new tree than the seeds which fall from the dry cones.

New sequoias grow only from seeds. When a seedling does take root, it often dies from <u>drought</u> and lack of light. But a few survive. So, every seed the chickaree drops from its perch high in the tree adds to the chance that one more sequoia might take root and live.

Thus, the eating habits of this squirrel help to keep these forest giants alive. It is playing an important role. The chickaree makes sure there will be new sequoia seeds sprouting up each year.

?

		Possible Score	Your Score

1. This passage talks about the Sequoia Cone-Cutter and its

    ☐ a. nest.
    ☐ b. appearance.
    ☐ c. eating habits.
    ☐ d. enemies.

    (15) ◯

2. Sequoias grow only from

    ☐ a. the trunk of living trees.
    ☐ b. roots.
    ☐ c. stumps.
    ☐ d. seeds.

    (15) ◯

3. Without the chickaree's help

    ☐ a. the tree would become diseased.
    ☐ b. bigger animals would attack the tree.
    ☐ c. sequoias might die out altogether.
    ☐ d. the sequoias would be killed by insects.

    (15) ◯

4. Which of the following describes the sequoia tree?

    ☐ a. Delicate
    ☐ b. Huge
    ☐ c. Weak
    ☐ d. Tiny

    (15) ◯

5. A <u>drought</u> is caused by

    ☐ a. too little sunshine.
    ☐ b. disease.
    ☐ c. lack of water.
    ☐ d. not enough food.

    (15) ◯

6. Main Idea

	Answer	Score
Mark the main idea	M	10
Mark the statement that is a detail	D	5
Mark the statement that is too narrow	N	5
Mark the statement that is too broad	B	5

a. The chickaree eats the outer part of the sequoia cone, but leaves the tiny seed.

b. The sequoia seeds are so small that it takes 1,200 of them to fill a teaspoon.

c. Living things often depend upon each other to survive.

d. The chickaree helps grow new sequoia trees by spreading the more fertile seeds.

Total Comprehension Score
(Add your scores and enter the total on the graph on page 103.)

Categories of Comprehension Questions

No. 1: Subject Matter	No. 4: Clarifying Devices
No. 2: Supporting Details	No. 5: Vocabulary in Context
No. 3: Conclusion	No. 6: Main Idea

14. The Kingfisher

What a handsome bird! With his bright blue "suit," white "vest," and wide, snowy "collar" he looks as if he's all dressed up to go to a party. But wait a minute! Who messed up his "hair"? The kingfisher's shaggy crest looks just a little odd with the rest of his neat appearance.

This bright-eyed fellow is about ten inches (about 25.4 centimeters) long and has a rather short neck, but why such a large bill for his small size? Birds that dive into the water to catch their food must have a long, strong bill to scoop up the fish.

The kingfisher is a remarkable fisher! He perches beside the river where he lives and waits for a fish to appear near the surface of the water. When he spots one, he bobs his head up and down and then flies out over the water. He pauses just an instant over his victim, takes aim and then SWOOPS down for his meal.

A kingfisher does not dive very deep, but it does usually go completely under the water. It pops back up to the surface instantly, and with a strong push with its wings it is back in the air again. Flying straight to the nearest rock, the kingfisher beats the fish to death against it and then gulps it down whole, headfirst — unless of course, there are baby "fishers" to be fed.

At the nesting site, the mother lays six to seven white eggs. She guards them carefully for about twenty-four days until they hatch. The female kingfisher can be identified by the bright chestnut band across her chest.

The nest is usually dug in the side of a riverbank. The average nest tunnel is from seven to ten feet (about 2.1 to 3.1 meters) deep. Each time a parent arrives at the tunnel, another chick appears at the entrance. It seems that the chicks take turns being fed. By the time the young leave home, the nest is littered with the bones of fish.

Baby kingfishers stay in the nest for four weeks after hatching. They have to be big and strong enough to fly before they leave the nest, for their home is directly over the water! If they don't fly — they will probably drown.

Kingfishers live on rivers or along any little stream that has plenty of fish. Young kingfishers aren't taught to fish by their parents; they seem to know how on their first try.

Usually the rivers are low, and small fish are <u>plentiful</u> during the summer, which is when the young make their first attempts at fishing. Soon they become experts like their parents.

Look for the kingfisher the next time you go fishing. Better yet, listen for him. His call is a loud, dry rattle, which he "barks" out for no good reason. Just your being there is reason enough for him to really bawl you out. He's the *king* fisherman and nobody else should be trying to catch his fish!

_____ **?** _____

	Possible Score	Your Score

1. The kingfisher is a

   ☐ a. tropical bird.
   ☐ b. game bird.
   ☐ c. fresh water bird.
   ☐ d. song bird.

   (15)   ◯

2. The kingfisher usually nests

   ☐ a. in empty groundhog burrows.
   ☐ b. on rocky cliffs.
   ☐ c. on the side of a riverbank.
   ☐ d. near the seashore.

   (15)   ◯

3. Baby kingfishers eat

   ☐ a. snails.
   ☐ b. fish.
   ☐ c. seeds.
   ☐ d. insects.

   (15)   ◯

4. As the female kingfisher guards her eggs for the first 24 days, she could be described as

   ☐ a. careless and lazy.
   ☐ b. nervous and shy.
   ☐ c. cruel and selfish.
   ☐ d. patient and alert.

   (15)   ◯

5. The kingfisher usually nests near rivers where small fish are *plentiful*. As used here, *plentiful* means

   ☐ a. most of the fish are adults.
   ☐ b. there are a lot of fish.
   ☐ c. the fish are slowly dying.
   ☐ d. the fish are spawning.

   (15)   ◯

6. Main Idea

	Answer	Score
Mark the main idea	M	10
Mark the statement that is a detail	D	5
Mark the statement that is too narrow	N	5
Mark the statement that is too broad	B	5

a. The kingfisher swoops down on fish from the air.

b. The kingfisher is an expert fisher.

c. Some birds can catch their own fish.

d. The eggs of the kingfisher take 24 days to hatch.

Total Comprehension Score
(Add your scores and enter the total on the graph on page 103.)

Categories of Comprehension Questions

No. 1: Subject Matter	No. 4: Clarifying Devices
No. 2: Supporting Details	No. 5: Vocabulary in Context
No. 3: Conclusion	No. 6: Main Idea

15. A Fish Fit for Emperors

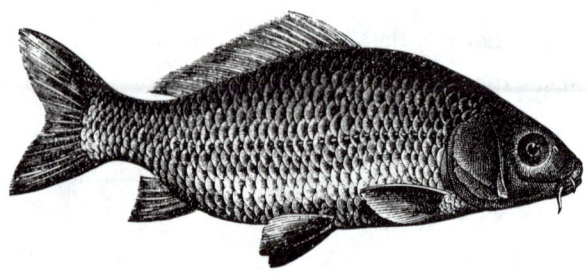

Years ago carp lived only in Asia. There they graced the private fishponds of emperors. They were eaten only on festive days. Then Europeans brought them to their countries where the carp was again the choice fare of kings. Monks kept them in monastery ponds. The monks fed them kitchen scraps. In England Izaak Walton, the patron of sport fishing, picked carp as one of the best fish. "The carp is the queen of rivers: a stately, good and very subtle fish," he wrote in *The Compleat Angler*. "And . . . if you fish for carp, you must put on a very large measure of patience."

Most Americans do not like carp, but Europeans are fond of them. Carp fishers in England go at their sport with great care and caution. They make many of our best trout fishers look unskilled. Careful carp fishers never touch bait with bare hands. They wear shoes with rubber soles and put sacks or heavy socks over the shoes to deaden the noise still more. Sometimes they cover their faces with bee veils or daub them with mud. This is because they know that a carp spooks quickly at the sight of a white face.

In England, any carp weighing more than ten pounds (about 45.4 kilograms) is classed as big. If fishers make catches weighing twenty pounds (about 9.07 kilograms) or more, they promptly hasten to taxidermists to have the prizes mounted. Then they display them proudly over their fireplaces, in their dens or at their offices. They talk about it for the rest of their lives.

Rarely, carp will take manmade lures, but mostly they are fished for with natural baits. There are many kinds from which to select. Expert carp fishers put on just enough bait to hide the tip of the hook because carp like small morsels.

A hooked carp moves like an express train! If the fisher is using a heavy line and rod, the catch can be drawn in at once. But with light tackle, the fun of a fight is ahead. Sometimes the carp will head for deep water to sulk. More often it'll whirl into the nearest weed bed. With a thin line or a light leader as the only hold on the carp, skillful handling is needed to keep the fish in clear water.

_____ **?** _____

	Possible Score	Your Score

1. What would be another good title for this passage?

   ☐ a. The Carp Family
   ☐ b. Nesting Habits of the Carp
   ☐ c. Carp and Trout Lures
   ☐ d. Fishing for Carp   (15)   ( )

2. Carp originally came from

   ☐ a. India.
   ☐ b. Africa.
   ☐ c. Europe.
   ☐ d. Asia.   (15)   ( )

3. The carp seems to be a favorite of English fishers because it is

   ☐ a. full of fight when hooked.
   ☐ b. a shy and lethargic fish.
   ☐ c. very rare.
   ☐ d. easy to catch.   (15)   ( )

4. A hooked carp moves like an express train. This means it

   ☐ a. travels in a slow, easy fashion.
   ☐ b. moves very fast.
   ☐ c. makes many stops.
   ☐ d. makes loud noises.   (15)   ( )

5. A good synonym for <u>hastens</u> is

   ☐ a. hurries.
   ☐ b. covers.
   ☐ c. hires.
   ☐ d. frightens.   (15)   ( )

6. Main Idea

	Answer	Score
Mark the main idea	M	10
Mark the statement that is a detail	D	5
Mark the statement that is too narrow	N	5
Mark the statement that is too broad	B	5

a. Some fish are harder to catch than others.

b. Catching carp requires a high level of care, caution and skill.

c. Expert carp fishers put on just enough bait to hide the hook tip.

d. Carp were once eaten only on festive days.

Total Comprehension Score
(Add your scores and enter the total on the graph on page 103.)

Categories of Comprehension Questions

No. 1: Subject Matter	No. 4: Clarifying Devices
No. 2: Supporting Details	No. 5: Vocabulary in Context
No. 3: Conclusion	No. 6: Main Idea

16. The Eider Duck

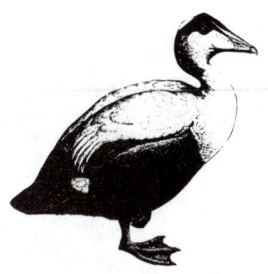

Children in Iceland sleep at night under *eiderdowns* (EYE der downs). These are quilts so light and soft that they almost seem to float above the bed. Eiderdowns are filled with the fine gray down of the common eider. This is a duck which lives along the coasts of the North Atlantic.

Common eiders nest in flocks on the islands around Iceland and along the fiords. Fiords are narrow inlets of the sea between cliffs.

In early May the common eiders come ashore in pairs. The <u>drab</u>, brown females pick the nest sites. They may either use last year's nest or make a new hollow in the sandy soil. They line them with bits of moss and grass. As soon as the females lay their eggs, they pull some down from their breasts to make a soft lining in the nest.

For the first ten days or so after the eggs are laid, the male sits quietly nearby. The female sits on the nest. Common eiders do not eat during this time, but they do drink. Every so often the male becomes restless. He stands up, moves about and then starts walking toward a freshwater pond nearby. The female, after covering the eggs with the down in the nest, follows him.

Once on the pond they swim, bathe and drink. But they never stay long. In a few minutes the female returns to her nest.

Back at the nest, she pulls the down away from the gray-green eggs with her bill. She settles down to another long stretch of incubation.

Icelanders who are lucky enough to have colonies of common eiders on their land take good care of the areas. They want the birds to come back year after year. They grade the land in broad ridges and dig a few hollows in the ground to attract the eiders.

Farmers collect the down from the nests three times each season. Twice in the early stages of incubation they take part of the down from each nest while the female duck is away. When they do this, they are careful not to take all the down. If they do, the female will leave the eggs and not come back. They often replace the down they take with soft moss and bits of grass. When the female returns, she will pluck more down from her breast to cushion the eggs.

After the young ducks leave, the farmers make a final round, taking all the down that is left. They must dry and clean the down before they send it to the market. The down from the common eider is gray fuzz. It is the lightest and softest material we know.

_____ ? _____

	Possible Score	Your Score
1. This passage tells us mostly about		
☐ a. the eating habits of the eider. ☐ b. the down of the eider. ☐ c. pollution and the eider duck. ☐ d. male eiders.	15	◯
2. The eider duck begins to nest in		
☐ a. late March. ☐ b. mid-April. ☐ c. early May. ☐ d. late June.	15	◯
3. Eider ducks		
☐ a. will soon become extinct. ☐ b. sometimes return to the same nest year after year. ☐ c. will begin to migrate in future years. ☐ d. are quarrelsome and do not get along with each other.	15	◯
4. An eiderdown quilt would feel		
☐ a. moist. ☐ b. soft. ☐ c. harsh. ☐ d. stiff.	15	◯
5. A good synonym for <u>drab</u> would be		
☐ a. dull. ☐ b. friendly. ☐ c. colorful. ☐ d. dawdle.	15	◯

6. Main Idea

	Answer	Score
Mark the main idea	M	10
Mark the statement that is a detail	D	5
Mark the statement that is too narrow	N	5
Mark the statement that is too broad	B	5

a. For the first 10 days after the eggs are laid, the parent eiders do not eat.

b. Some natural materials are very soft and therefore useful to humans.

c. The down from the eider duck, the lightest and fluffiest material known, is collected to make quilts.

d. The down from the common eider is collected 3 times a season from the eider nest.

Total Comprehension Score
(Add your scores and enter the total on the graph on page 103.)

Categories of Comprehension Questions

No. 1: Subject Matter	No. 4: Clarifying Devices
No. 2: Supporting Details	No. 5: Vocabulary in Context
No. 3: Conclusion	No. 6: Main Idea

17. Bats Keep Their Ears Clean

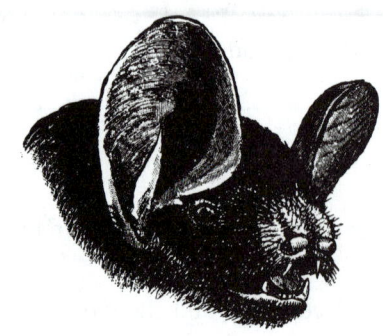

Animals keep themselves clean in different ways. Dogs usually get clean by scratching themselves. This gets rid of the loose hairs. They don't take a water bath often — on their own anyway. Too much water makes a dog's skin dry out, and it may crack.

When children take baths, they sometimes forget to clean their ears. But bats don't forget. Their ears must always be clean because bats find their way by listening to sounds.

A bat puts the thumb of its winged front "hand" in its ear and twists it around and around to loosen the dirt. The rest of its body is kept spotless with its long, pink tongue.

A jackrabbit also remembers to clean its ears. It pushes them forward with a foot, so its tongue can reach them. It cleans its feet by shaking each one to loosen the dirt and then licking it.

Squirrels are mostly concerned with cleaning their tails. They spend hours grooming their tails, but for good reason. A squirrel's tail acts as a parachute when it jumps and as a "balancing pole" when it runs along branches. In winter, asleep in its nest, it wraps itself in a warm tail "blanket."

Just as people use combs to keep their hair smooth, so do many animals. After bathing, the duckbill platypus combs its fur with a long claw until it's smooth and in place.

Bears use claw "combs" too. They sharpen their claws on stumps and tree trunks. This keeps their "combs" sharp. Claws are also the bear's main weapons of defense.

All of Mother Nature's animals know that keeping clean is a must for survival.

?

	Possible Score	Your Score

1. This passage tells us mostly about how some animals

   ☐ a. move by sound.
   ☐ b. wash their food.
   ☐ c. keep their bodies clean.
   ☐ d. sharpen their claws.

   (15)   ○

2. Bats find their way by

   ☐ a. listening to sounds.
   ☐ b. feeling things around them.
   ☐ c. guesswork.
   ☐ d. tasting the air.

   (15)   ○

3. We can see that

   ☐ a. not all animals keep clean by using water.
   ☐ b. animals don't clean themselves very often.
   ☐ c. teeth are a bear's only weapon.
   ☐ d. most animals wash their food regularly.

   (15)   ○

4. A squirrel uses its tail for

   ☐ a. fighting.
   ☐ b. warmth.
   ☐ c. nesting material.
   ☐ d. hiding.

   (15)   ○

5. As used in this passage <u>spotless</u> means

   ☐ a. dry.
   ☐ b. oiled.
   ☐ c. wet.
   ☐ d. clean.

   (15)   ○

73

6. Main Idea

	Answer	Score
Mark the main idea	M	10
Mark the statement that is a detail	D	5
Mark the statement that is too narrow	N	5
Mark the statement that is too broad	B	5

a. Animals keep themselves clean in several ways.

b. Too much water makes a dog's skin dry out.

c. Animals groom their ears and fur in several ways.

d. Dogs clean their fur by scratching themselves.

Total Comprehension Score
(Add your scores and enter the total on the graph on page 103.)

Categories of Comprehension Questions

No. 1: Subject Matter	No. 4: Clarifying Devices
No. 2: Supporting Details	No. 5: Vocabulary in Context
No. 3: Conclusion	No. 6: Main Idea

18. From Fawn to Yearling

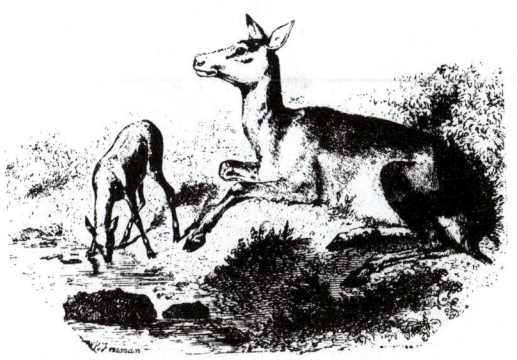

The doe will go just far enough away so that she can still see her babies or hear them if they should cry out. A young fawn bleats almost like a baby lamb. If danger comes near the fawns, the mother will attempt to lure it away by showing herself. In some cases, if the danger is from a small animal, such as a dog, the doe may try to drive it away. Does have been known to kill snakes that crawled near their fawns. A mother deer's sharp hooves are very <u>effective</u> weapons.

The doe will come back to the fawns four or five times a day to allow them to nurse. The fawns can drink eight ounces (about 236.6 milliliters) of milk in less than a minute. After the fawns have nursed, they lie down and the doe leaves them again. Occasionally the fawns try to follow their mother. One doe that I was watching had trouble with a fawn that wanted to follow her. Finally, she took one of her front feet and, putting it across the baby's back, pressed until the little one lay down. Then she left to find food for herself or to rest.

After four or five days, the fawn's hoofs, which were soft at birth, begin to dry and harden. By the time the fawn is three weeks old, it is big and strong enough to be able to accompany the doe when she feeds.

This is when the fawn starts to wean itself. Imitating its mother, the fawn nibbles at a piece of grass or shrub or other vegetation. As it develops a taste for plant material, it gradually eats more. With its stomach partially filled with plant food, the fawn requires less milk. In a short time the fawn will be weaned completely and will eat only foliage.

All deer, young and old alike, have bright, reddish brown hair in the summertime. It is thin and solid and provides protection against insects. In September all deer shed their summer coats and get their brand-new winter coats. The winter hair is long, kinky, hollow and filled with air. This coat keeps the deer snug and warm. It is at this time that the fawns begin to look exactly like miniature adult deer.

The spotted fawns quickly grow to be like their mother or father. As a yearling, each will wander through the woods alone, now able to take care of itself.

_____ **?** _____

	Possible Score	Your Score

1. What would be another good title for this passage?

    ☐ a. Growing Up
    ☐ b. Storing Food Is Fun
    ☐ c. Deer Season Is Open
    ☐ d. How To Track a Deer

    15

2. What does a mother deer use to protect her young?

    ☐ a. Her tremendous size
    ☐ b. A foul odor
    ☐ c. Her sharp teeth
    ☐ d. Her hoofs

    15

3. After reading this passage, we can see that white tail deer feed on

    ☐ a. carrion.
    ☐ b. plants.
    ☐ c. insects.
    ☐ d. meat.

    15

4. The writer compares a fawn to a lamb in order to compare

    ☐ a. the look-alike appearance of each.
    ☐ b. their sizes and sharp hearing.
    ☐ c. the similar sounds they make.
    ☐ d. their appetites.

    15

5. An <u>effective</u> weapon is

    ☐ a. harmless.
    ☐ b. unnecessary.
    ☐ c. broken.
    ☐ d. useful.

    15

6. Main Idea

	Answer	Score
Mark the main idea	M	10
Mark the statement that is a detail	D	5
Mark the statement that is too narrow	N	5
Mark the statement that is too broad	B	5

a. A fawn learns to eat plant food by copying its mother's feeding habits.

b. Many animals are taught how to survive by their mothers.

c. A fawn depends on its mother at first but quickly learns to take care of itself.

d. The fawn's hoofs begin to dry and harden after 4 to 5 days.

Total Comprehension Score
(Add your scores and enter the total on the graph on page 103.)

Categories of Comprehension Questions

No. 1: Subject Matter	No. 4: Clarifying Devices
No. 2: Supporting Details	No. 5: Vocabulary in Context
No. 3: Conclusion	No. 6: Main Idea

19. Mischief-Makers

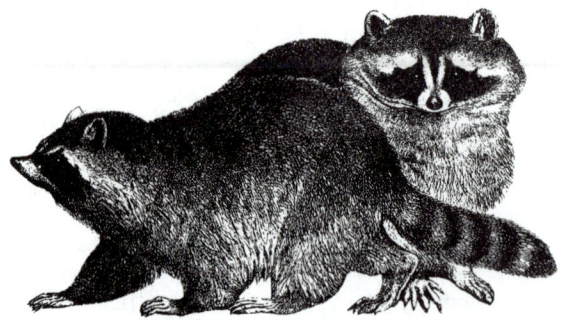

The common raccoon is found in North America and Central America. It is not found wild in other parts of the world. Like people, it can live in almost every part of this country. It is found from coast to coast.

Full-grown raccoons weigh about 25 pounds (about 11.3 kilograms). In April or May the female has her young — usually four to six in a litter. Their eyes are closed when they are born, and they are helpless. But they seem to be already dressed for a Halloween party. They have their fur coats on and black masks across their faces.

For their first ten weeks, the young raccoons stay home, usually in a hollow tree, waiting for their mothers to come back and nurse them. Their father does not stay around or help with raising them. Then during the last part of summer, the young ones follow their mother out of the hollow tree at night and begin learning to hunt for their own food.

Sometimes they catch frogs and crayfish from the creek. Or they may search for turtle eggs, insects and now and then a farmer's chicken. They are very fond of beechnuts and acorns. When growing corn begins to get sweet, the raccoons feast on it. The next day the farmer knows this when it's clear that the corn is gone, and there are animal tracks in the soft earth. This is one reason why raccoons are called "mischief-makers."

Dogs are the raccoon's enemies and will drive them into trees. If the dogs catch them, they sometimes kill the raccoons. But raccoons are good fighters, too. Sometimes the raccoon will lead an old hound into the water, jump on its head and hold it under until it drowns. One raccoon, chased by five big hounds, finally grew tired of the chase and stopped to fight. It whipped them all!

_____ **?** _____

| | Possible Score | Your Score |

1. What would be another good title for this passage?

   ☐ a. Raccoons and Chipmunks
   ☐ b. The Coonskin Cap
   ☐ c. A Good Pet
   ☐ d. The Common Raccoon

   (15)

2. Raccoons usually build their nests in

   ☐ a. thickets.
   ☐ b. burrows.
   ☐ c. rock shelters.
   ☐ d. hollow trees.

   (15)

3. Raccoons are mostly active

   ☐ a. during the day.
   ☐ b. at night.
   ☐ c. when temperatures are warm.
   ☐ d. in rainy weather.

   (15)

4. In the last paragraph, the raccoon could be described as

   ☐ a. curious.
   ☐ b. a brave fighter.
   ☐ c. mean.
   ☐ d. shy and bashful.

   (15)

5. Raccoons are <u>fond</u> of beechnuts. This means they

   ☐ a. hide them.
   ☐ b. throw them away.
   ☐ c. like them.
   ☐ d. wash them.

   (15)

6. Main Idea

	Answer	Score
Mark the main idea	M	10
Mark the statement that is a detail	D	5
Mark the statement that is too narrow	N	5
Mark the statement that is too broad	B	5

a. There are usually 4 to 6 baby raccoons to a litter.

b. Baby raccoons are found in deep woods where there are hollow trees.

c. Many interesting creatures are found over a wide area.

d. The raccoon is an interesting animal found in North and Central America.

Total Comprehension Score
(Add your scores and enter the total on the graph on page 103.)

Categories of Comprehension Questions

No. 1: Subject Matter	No. 4: Clarifying Devices
No. 2: Supporting Details	No. 5: Vocabulary in Context
No. 3: Conclusion	No. 6: Main Idea

20. Getting Ready To Fly

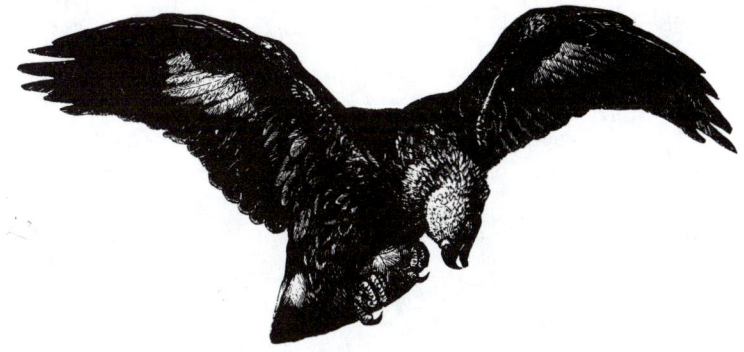

Close to three months old the eaglet did a "dance." This is the dance it will use later when it corners prey for its food. As I watched it, I saw that it often stared at a piece of rabbit meat. Then it would lean forward as if to take flight before jumping on it. It would grasp it and tear it with its beak and hop around the edge of the nest.

When the eaglet was just past three months old, it stood on the edge of the cliff and looked toward the valley floor. It was ready for its first flight. For the first time, the young golden eagle left the nest.

Unlike the bald eagle, whose main food is fish, this golden eagle will feed mostly on prairie dogs, rabbits and ground squirrels. It will seldom eat something that it has not killed itself.

As I stood watching the young eagle in flight, I knew that humans would be its only real enemy. Sometimes people shoot it as a killer of other animals. This is against the law because the golden eagle is not a pest. Its prey is mostly small animals which harm crops. It is also in danger because of the <u>pesticides</u> humans use on crops to kill insects. The poisons can build up in plant-eating animals. They will then be passed on to the eagle that eats them.

I watched as the strong, young eagle faded into the sky. I thought about the many adventures and the many dangers the future held for it.

?

1. This passage is talking about

    - [ ] a. a young eagle.
    - [ ] b. how eagles mate.
    - [ ] c. catching eagles.
    - [ ] d. where eagles live.

2. How old is the eaglet?

    - [ ] a. 1 week
    - [ ] b. 3 weeks
    - [ ] c. 3 months
    - [ ] d. 4 months

3. The writer suggests that eagles can be poisoned by

    - [ ] a. drinking polluted water.
    - [ ] b. eating plants.
    - [ ] c. the animals they eat.
    - [ ] d. catching fish.

4. The third paragraph tells us that the golden eagle and the bald eagle differ in

    - [ ] a. size.
    - [ ] b. diet.
    - [ ] c. color.
    - [ ] d. personality.

5. Which of the following describes pesticides?

    - [ ] a. Plants
    - [ ] b. Poisons
    - [ ] c. Animals
    - [ ] d. Insects

6. Main Idea

	Answer	Score
Mark the main idea	M	10
Mark the statement that is a detail	D	5
Mark the statement that is too narrow	N	5
Mark the statement that is too broad	B	5

a. The young eaglet learns to fly, but there are many dangers in the future.

b. The eaglet practices before it takes its first real flight.

c. It is against the law to shoot eagles, for they are not pests.

d. The skills of animals cannot always protect them.

Total Comprehension Score
(Add your scores and enter the total on the graph on page 103.)

Categories of Comprehension Questions

No. 1: Subject Matter	No. 4: Clarifying Devices
No. 2: Supporting Details	No. 5: Vocabulary in Context
No. 3: Conclusion	No. 6: Main Idea

21. The Engelmann Spruce

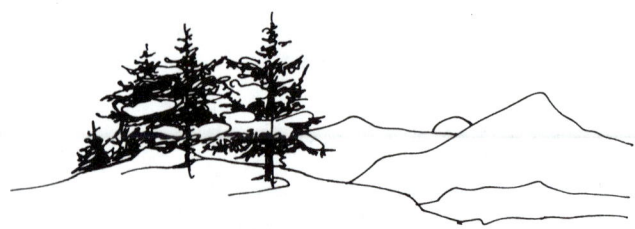

Engelmann spruce trees are *conifers* (trees which have cones). They are one of the world's toughest kinds of tree. They can survive the severe weather high up a mountainside.

As on most evergreen trees, the cones are strong to protect the fragile seeds inside. Each needle is covered with thick wax. This helps keep it from losing its moisture in the cold, dry wind.

In the autumn, fertile seeds are dropped from the cones. As they fall, the wind sweeps them away. The wind doesn't care where it drops the seeds. Many come to rest on rocks or at the bottom of an alpine lake, where they die.

Some seeds land on open ground. Yet, they often die before the end of the first winter. Those which happen to land behind rocks or in a place where other Engelmann are growing may live. There are thousands of seeds produced. But only a few land where the spring thaw will help them sprout.

During the short alpine summer, a spruce seed sends out roots and a very tiny shoot about a quarter-inch (about 6.4 millimeters) tall. But the winter will come soon with temperatures that often drop to minus 50° Fahrenheit (minus 45° Celsius). Its force will be strong and its damage great. Even the spring thaw can be harmful. A spring landslide may tear a young seedling from its new home.

Where there is some shelter and the right amount of heat, rain and light, the young Engelmann spruce will keep growing, but very, very slowly. After five years, it may be only three-fourths of an inch (about 19.1 millimeters) tall. It may keep growing for 300 years, but it will never grow very tall. The strong wind and bitter cold will kill any limbs that try to grow straight up. Only those that grow along the ground and away from the wind will survive. A few trees have survived the wind and cold for as long as 500 years. These old trees have grown into strange shapes.

Tragedy can still come quickly in the alpine forest, even to a tree which has weathered 500 winters. A fire can kill in ten minutes what took nature centuries to build. After a fire, the tree's green beauty is gone. Only a burned-out trunk remains.

But even in death the tree is important to alpine life. Its black body blocks the wind and provides new seedlings with shelter in which to grow. Maybe among them will be a tree able to take the dead tree's place. It might survive the harsh life of the mountains.

?

| | Possible Score | Your Score |

1. This passage is about the Engelmann Spruce and

   ☐ a. uses of its bark.
   ☐ b. its root system.
   ☐ c. its unusual color.
   ☐ d. how it grows.

   15

2. A conifer is a tree that

   ☐ a. changes color.
   ☐ b. has cones.
   ☐ c. loses its leaves.
   ☐ d. does not need sunlight.

   15

3. This passage hints that evergreen trees have strong cones so that

   ☐ a. the seeds will not be harmed.
   ☐ b. water will not be lost.
   ☐ c. animals will not eat them.
   ☐ d. the seeds will not grow.

   15

4. An "alpine forest" is found

   ☐ a. near the seashore.
   ☐ b. on level plains.
   ☐ c. high in the mountains.
   ☐ d. in the middle of a desert.

   15

5. A <u>severe</u> winter is very

   ☐ a. harsh.
   ☐ b. warm.
   ☐ c. rainy.
   ☐ d. sunny.

   15

6. Main Idea

	Answer	Score
Mark the main idea	M	10
Mark the statement that is a detail	D	5
Mark the statement that is too narrow	N	5
Mark the statement that is too broad	B	5

a. The Engelmann spruce is one of the world's toughest trees.

b. Some trees can survive extremely harsh conditions.

c. After 5 years, the Engelmann spruce may be only ¾-inch (about 19.1 millimeters) tall.

d. The Engelmann spruce has to withstand temperatures of minus 50 degrees Fahrenheit (minus 45° Celsius).

Total Comprehension Score
(Add your scores and enter the total on the graph on page 103.)

Categories of Comprehension Questions

No. 1: Subject Matter	No. 4: Clarifying Devices
No. 2: Supporting Details	No. 5: Vocabulary in Context
No. 3: Conclusion	No. 6: Main Idea

22. The Game of Sticks

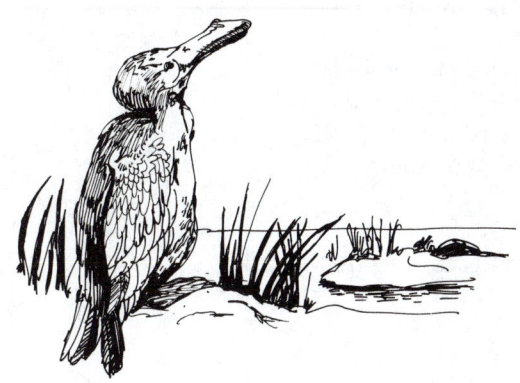

The spoonbill must live in areas where food is easy to find. These places are called *food niches*. A good food niche for the spoonbill is a tidal pool. Here ocean water mixes with fresh stream water. These pools are only three to four inches (about 7.6 to 10.1 centimeters) deep. They are breeding places for sea life and are alive with minnows, insects and crabs.

Spoonbills are easy to recognize. Roseate spoonbills stand two and a half feet (about .75 meters) high. They have a wing spread of four feet (about 1.2 meters) or more. In flight their legs and long necks are outstretched.

Many times during the nesting season a whole flock of spoonbills will take flight just after feeding. Soon, as if on signal, they drift down. Then they stand motionless for an hour or so with their beaks pointing to the sky. Naturalists cannot explain why they "skygaze" like this.

The male spoonbill courts a female in a game of "sticks" while other spoonbills look on. An adult male picks up a stick and rattles it in his bill so that it clatters. The female ignores him until he struts closer to her. Then she watches him closely as he wags his head and waves the stick. Suddenly, he drops it at her feet and steps back. If she picks up the stick, it means she accepts him for her mate. For a moment she pauses, then quickly takes up the stick in her bill. The stick will be the first of dozens they will weave together to make a nest for the eggs. The male joins her on her perch, and together they jump down and walk away. The flock, which has been watching, bow heads low as the pair strolls by.

Today there is less danger of extinction for the spoonbills. Under the protection of the Everglades National Park, the red birds have increased in number. Here they no longer need fear that people will harm them.

_____ ? _____

	Possible Score	Your Score

1. This passage is mainly about

   ☐ a. the spoonbill's mating habits.
   ☐ b. how spoonbills survive the winter.
   ☐ c. the enemies of the spoonbill.
   ☐ d. how to find spoonbills.

   15

2. Areas where food is easy to find is called a food

   ☐ a. clutch.
   ☐ b. niche.
   ☐ c. notch.
   ☐ d. chain.

   15

3. We can see that the spoonbill

   ☐ a. now has a better chance at survival.
   ☐ b. will soon become extinct.
   ☐ c. is being bred for its feathers.
   ☐ d. is killing too much sea life.

   15

4. The fourth paragraph discusses the spoonbill's

   ☐ a. survival habits.
   ☐ b. mating habits.
   ☐ c. migratory habits.
   ☐ d. eating habits.

   15

5. A <u>motionless</u> spoonbill stands

   ☐ a. on one foot.
   ☐ b. on its head.
   ☐ c. perfectly still.
   ☐ d. in the water.

   15

6. Main Idea

	Answer	Score
Mark the main idea	M	10
Mark the statement that is a detail	D	5
Mark the statement that is too narrow	N	5
Mark the statement that is too broad	B	5

a. Many shore birds have interesting habits.

b. The spoonbill is a shore bird of peculiar nesting and mating habits.

c. The spoonbill finds a mate with a game of sticks.

d. Spoonbills are 2½ feet (about .75 meters) tall with a wingspan of over 4 feet (about 1.2 meters).

Total Comprehension Score
(Add your scores and enter the total on the graph on page 103.)

Categories of Comprehension Questions

No. 1: Subject Matter	No. 4: Clarifying Devices
No. 2: Supporting Details	No. 5: Vocabulary in Context
No. 3: Conclusion	No. 6: Main Idea

23. Our Grasslands

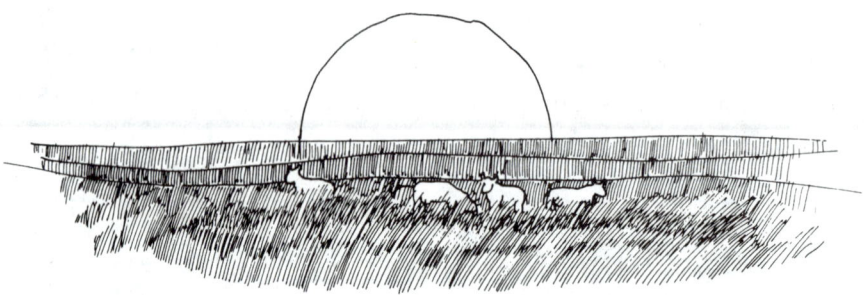

One hundred and fifty years ago great numbers of bison, pronghorn, turkey, quail and other wildlife roamed our prairies. They ate the wild grass that covered millions of acres with a thick, tough <u>sod</u>.

As settlers moved west, they brought herds of cattle and sheep. These grass eaters also fed on the ranges. Soon there was not enough food for them and for the wild animals as well.

Pioneers killed the wild animals for meat and skins. This left the grass for livestock. Huge cattle herds ate more and more of the grass. As they were driven to market, they trampled and damaged the grasslands.

In 1881 the United States Congress passed the Homestead Act. This gave 160 acres (about 64 hectares) of land to anyone who would live on it, plow it and plant crops. Homesteaders plowed the sod and planted wheat and other grains. More of the grasslands were destroyed.

These new crops grew well in many places, but sometimes there was not enough water for grain. The sod that had soaked up rain like a sponge and had held the water was now gone. Topsoil washed away when it rained. Then it dried and blew away with the prairie winds.

At last, people saw the importance of the grasslands. They knew that they must do something to stop the destruction of it. For the past fifty years, a science called *range management* has helped save and improve these grasslands.

Fine natural grasslands are now on the increase. Many plowed fields have gone back to grass. Grass is the best crop for restoring land that has been worn out by other crops or by overgrazing.

Grass is also the cheapest known food for cattle and sheep. And it is one of the best for them. But care is now taken to limit the number of cattle or sheep which graze on a certain field. With less livestock per field, some of each grass plant is left after grazing. This part of the plant will grow again and make seeds for new grass.

?

	Possible Score	Your Score

1. This passage is mainly about

   ☐ a. wetlands.
   ☐ b. forests.
   ☐ c. prairies.
   ☐ d. deserts.

   (15) ○

2. In 1881 the United States Congress passed the

   ☐ a. Intolerable Acts.
   ☐ b. Homestead Act.
   ☐ c. Monroe Doctrine.
   ☐ d. Civil Rights Act.

   (15) ○

3. The grasslands

   ☐ a. were wastelands.
   ☐ b. supported very little life.
   ☐ c. held the soil together.
   ☐ d. are dry and hot.

   (15) ○

4. The writer feels that the grasslands should be

   ☐ a. eliminated.
   ☐ b. flooded.
   ☐ c. replaced.
   ☐ d. protected.

   (15) ○

5. Another word for <u>sod</u> is

   ☐ a. meat.
   ☐ b. underbrush.
   ☐ c. turf.
   ☐ d. gullies.

   (15) ○

6. Main Idea

	Answer	Score
Mark the main idea	M	10
Mark the statement that is a detail	D	5
Mark the statement that is too narrow	N	5
Mark the statement that is too broad	B	5

a. The settlers grazed too many cattle on the grasslands.

b. People have learned to use natural resources carefully.

c. The grasslands, once destroyed by overgrazing and farming, are being restored.

d. The sod of the United States grasslands soaked up rain like a sponge and then held it.

Total Comprehension Score
(Add your scores and enter the total on the graph on page 103.)

Categories of Comprehension Questions

No. 1: Subject Matter	No. 4: Clarifying Devices
No. 2: Supporting Details	No. 5: Vocabulary in Context
No. 3: Conclusion	No. 6: Main Idea

24. The White-Footed Mouse and Its Young

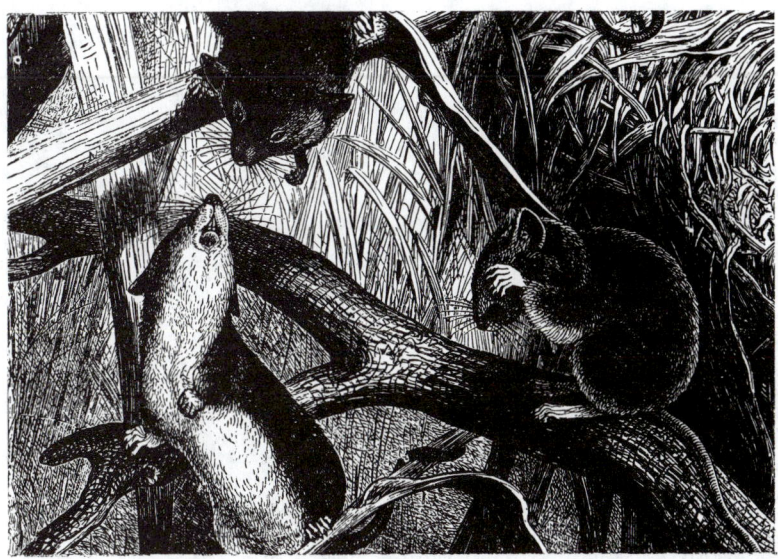

Life is good for young, white-footed mice. They enjoy the warmth, safety and nourishment of their mother. In a few weeks, they will be forced to leave the nest to make room for a new litter. In eight weeks, they could have litters of their own. Until then, though, devoted care is lavished upon them by their mother.

Before their birth, the female shares with her chosen mate the domestic duty of finding just the perfect nest. They then weave into it blades of dry grass and leaves and line it with bark. But just before giving birth, the female evicts the male.

When the young are a few days old, the female lets the male rejoin his family. Both parents wash their delicate young, licking each of them gently until all are spotless. The male is then sent out to find food for his mate while she nurses and warms her brood.

In three or four weeks, the young mice will be on their own. They will have to find their own food. They eat rotten acorns, new grass and insect eggs from the woodlands near the nest.

If they live long enough, their furry backs will turn from gray to brown. But their survival will be difficult. Larger animals will be a constant threat. Owls, hawks, crows and other birds will wait to swoop down on them. The average white-foot survives only one year.

But when they are young, hunger, cold and death are far away. The only reality is their mother's care — round-the-clock care found only at home.

		Possible Score	Your Score

1. This passage deals mostly with

   ☐ a. young mice.
   ☐ b. the mating of white-footed mice.
   ☐ c. duties of the male white-footed mouse.
   ☐ d. the hibernation of mice.

   15

2. The life expectancy of the white-footed mouse is

   ☐ a. 8 weeks.
   ☐ b. 6 months.
   ☐ c. 1 year.
   ☐ d. 2 years.

   15

3. We can guess that the white-footed mouse is easy prey for

   ☐ a. the domestic dog.
   ☐ b. raccoons.
   ☐ c. skunks.
   ☐ d. some birds.

   15

4. When the female mouse "nurses" her brood, she gives them

   ☐ a. a bath.
   ☐ b. food.
   ☐ c. a rest.
   ☐ d. shelter.

   15

5. The female <u>evicts</u> the male. This means the male has been

   ☐ a. killed.
   ☐ b. trapped.
   ☐ c. put out.
   ☐ d. wounded.

   15

6. Main Idea

	Answer	Score
Mark the main idea	M	10
Mark the statement that is a detail	D	5
Mark the statement that is too narrow	N	5
Mark the statement that is too broad	B	5

a. The female white-footed mouse looks for a perfect nest for her young.

b. Most mothers lavish care upon their young offspring.

c. The nest of the white-footed mouse is made of dry grass and leaves lined with bark.

d. For a few weeks, young white-footed mice receive the devoted care of their mother.

Total Comprehension Score
(Add your scores and enter the total on the graph on page 103.)

Categories of Comprehension Questions

No. 1: Subject Matter	No. 4: Clarifying Devices
No. 2: Supporting Details	No. 5: Vocabulary in Context
No. 3: Conclusion	No. 6: Main Idea

25. Codfish

Long ago, many large codfish could be found in the rich feeding grounds of the Grand Banks off Newfoundland. The Vikings caught these fish and traded their catch with the people of Europe. Then in the 1400s the Portuguese found the Grand Banks. And soon the French and English joined the Portuguese on these cod grounds.

Since there were so many fish and so few people, there were enough cod for all. Big fish produced up to nine million eggs each year. Even though only a few of these survived, there were always great numbers of cod in the North Atlantic.

Soon dried and salted codfish were feeding the settlers in North America. Codfish were being shipped all over the world. The oil of the cod's liver was used in medicines. Its air bladder was used to make glue. Almost every part of the fish was used.

Cod fishers sailed from their ports in handsome brigs and schooners. When they reached the fishing grounds, each fisher left the mother ship to sail off in a dory. They used long handlines with many hooks tied to them. Sometimes the ships fishing on the best grounds numbered in the hundreds. Even so, there were plenty of fish.

Then fishers changed their way of fishing on the Grand Banks. From Great Britain and Norway came the *otter trawl*. This is a large net with side panels. The panels keep the net's mouth open as it is dragged along the bottom. In this way, six people could catch in one hour what it might take sixty people *days* to catch with handlines.

These nets were first used in the Grand Banks around 1900. In thirty years, people saw that the trawlers were catching too many fish. They were not leaving enough grown-up cod to produce eggs and carry on the species. But the trawlers did not want to go back to the old ways. Cod were taken in huge numbers. Ten years later there were only a few fish left in grounds that had once contained thousands.

In the early 1970s, the many nations that fished for cod signed a treaty which limited the places to be fished and the size of the catch. This seems to be helping. It would be a worldwide tragedy if the cod should become scarce. Millions of people around the world depend on the codfish as their main food.

?

	Possible Score	Your Score

1. This passage talks mainly about the

   ☐ a. mating habits of the codfish.
   ☐ b. codfish family.
   ☐ c. uses of codfish oil.
   ☐ d. history of cod fishing.

   15

2. The Grand Banks are located off the coast of

   ☐ a. Florida.
   ☐ b. Newfoundland.
   ☐ c. Iceland.
   ☐ d. France.

   15

3. We can see that the early users of codfish were

   ☐ a. cheap.
   ☐ b. lively.
   ☐ c. not wasteful.
   ☐ d. careless.

   15

4. In this passage the mother ship is

   ☐ a. a ghost ship.
   ☐ b. the main ship.
   ☐ c. a small rowboat.
   ☐ d. the damaged ship.

   15

5. A <u>handsome</u> schooner is

   ☐ a. untidy and often dirty.
   ☐ b. pleasing to look at.
   ☐ c. not able to travel very fast.
   ☐ d. very large and awkward.

   15

6. Main Idea

	Answer	Score
Mark the main idea	M	10
Mark the statement that is a detail	D	5
Mark the statement that is too narrow	N	5
Mark the statement that is too broad	B	5

a. The use of otter nets has made codfish on the Grand Banks scarce.

b. With the otter net, codfish could be caught much quicker and easier.

c. The air bladder of the cod was used to make glue.

d. There are not so many codfish as there used to be.

Total Comprehension Score
(Add your scores and enter the total on the graph on page 103.)

Categories of Comprehension Questions

No. 1: Subject Matter	No. 4: Clarifying Devices
No. 2: Supporting Details	No. 5: Vocabulary in Context
No. 3: Conclusion	No. 6: Main Idea

Acknowledgments

The passages appearing in this book have been reprinted with the kind permission of the following publications and publishers to whom the author is indebted:

Aramco World Magazine, published by The Arabian American Oil Company, New York, New York.

The Communicator, published by the New York State Outdoor Education Association, Syracuse, New York.

The Conservationist, published by the New York State Conservation Department, Albany, New York.

A Cornell Science Leaflet, published by the New York State College of Agriculture and Life Sciences, a unit of the State University, at Cornell University, Ithaca, New York.

Food, The Yearbook of Agriculture, published by the United States Department of Agriculture, Washington, D.C.

Handbook of Nature-Study, published by Comstock Publishing Company, Ithaca, New York.

Kansas Fish & Game, published by the Kansas Forestry, Fish and Game Commission, Pratt, Kansas.

National Wildlife, published by The National Wildlife Federation, Washington, D.C.

Outdoor Oklahoma, published by the Oklahoma Department of Wildlife Conservation, Oklahoma City, Oklahoma.

Pennsylvania Game News, published by the Pennsylvania Game Commission, Harrisburg, Pennsylvania.

Ranger Rick's Nature Magazine, published by The National Wildlife Federation, Washington, D.C.

The Tennessee Conservationist, published by the Tennessee Department of Conservation and the Tennessee Game and Fish Commission.

Answer Key: Book 5

Passage 1:	1.c	2.a	3.a	4.b	5.c	6a.N	6b.M	6c.B	6d.D
Passage 2:	1.a	2.d	3.b	4.b	5.d	6a.N	6b.B	6c.M	6d.D
Passage 3:	1.b	2.a	3.d	4.c	5.a	6a.D	6b.N	6c.B	6d.M
Passage 4:	1.d	2.c	3.b	4.b	5.c	6a.M	6b.D	6c.B	6d.N
Passage 5:	1.b	2.b	3.d	4.a	5.d	6a.N	6b.M	6c.B	6d.D
Passage 6:	1.c	2.b	3.c	4.c	5.b	6a.M	6b.B	6c.N	6d.D
Passage 7:	1.a	2.c	3.a	4.c	5.d	6a.D	6b.B	6c.M	6d.N
Passage 8:	1.d	2.c	3.a	4.a	5.d	6a.B	6b.M	6c.D	6d.N
Passage 9:	1.c	2.b	3.d	4.d	5.a	6a.M	6b.B	6c.N	6d.D
Passage 10:	1.b	2.d	3.a	4.b	5.d	6a.N	6b.B	6c.D	6d.M
Passage 11:	1.a	2.d	3.a	4.a	5.c	6a.D	6b.N	6c.M	6d.B
Passage 12:	1.b	2.c	3.b	4.c	5.b	6a.B	6b.D	6c.M	6d.N
Passage 13:	1.c	2.d	3.c	4.b	5.c	6a.N	6b.D	6c.B	6d.M

Answer Key: Book 5

Passage 14:	1.c	2.c	3.b	4.d	5.b	6a.**N**	6b.**M**	6c.**B**	6d.**D**
Passage 15:	1.d	2.d	3.a	4.b	5.a	6a.**B**	6b.**M**	6c.**N**	6d.**D**
Passage 16:	1.b	2.c	3.b	4.b	5.a	6a.**D**	6b.**B**	6c.**M**	6d.**N**
Passage 17:	1.c	2.a	3.a	4.b	5.d	6a.**B**	6b.**D**	6c.**M**	6d.**N**
Passage 18:	1.a	2.d	3.b	4.c	5.d	6a.**N**	6b.**B**	6c.**M**	6d.**D**
Passage 19:	1.d	2.d	3.b	4.b	5.c	6a.**D**	6b.**N**	6c.**B**	6d.**M**
Passage 20:	1.a	2.c	3.c	4.b	5.b	6a.**M**	6b.**N**	6c.**D**	6d.**B**
Passage 21:	1.d	2.b	3.a	4.c	5.a	6a.**M**	6b.**B**	6c.**D**	6d.**N**
Passage 22:	1.a	2.b	3.a	4.b	5.c	6a.**B**	6b.**M**	6c.**N**	6d.**D**
Passage 23:	1.c	2.b	3.c	4.d	5.c	6a.**N**	6b.**B**	6c.**M**	6d.**D**
Passage 24:	1.a	2.c	3.d	4.b	5.c	6a.**N**	6b.**B**	6c.**D**	6d.**M**
Passage 25:	1.d	2.b	3.c	4.b	5.b	6a.**M**	6b.**N**	6c.**D**	6d.**B**

Diagnostic Chart (For Student Correction)

Directions: Write your final answers in the *upper* part of the passage block. Then correct your answers using the Answer Key on pages 100 and 101. If your answer is correct, do not make any more marks in the block. If your answer is incorrect, write the letter of the correct answer in the *lower* part of the block.

Categories of Comprehension Skills	Reading Passage 1 2 3 4 5 6 7 8 9 10 11 12 13 14 15 16 17 18 19 20 21 22 23 24 25
1. Subject Matter	
2. Supporting Details	
3. Conclusion	
4. Clarifying Devices	
5. Vocabulary in Context	
6. Main Idea — Main Idea	
Detail	
Too Narrow	
Too Broad	

Progress Graph

Directions: Write your Total Comprehension Score in the box under the number for each passage. Then put an *x* along the line above each box to show your Total Comprehension Score for that passage. Then make a graph of your progress. Draw a line to connect the *x*'s.

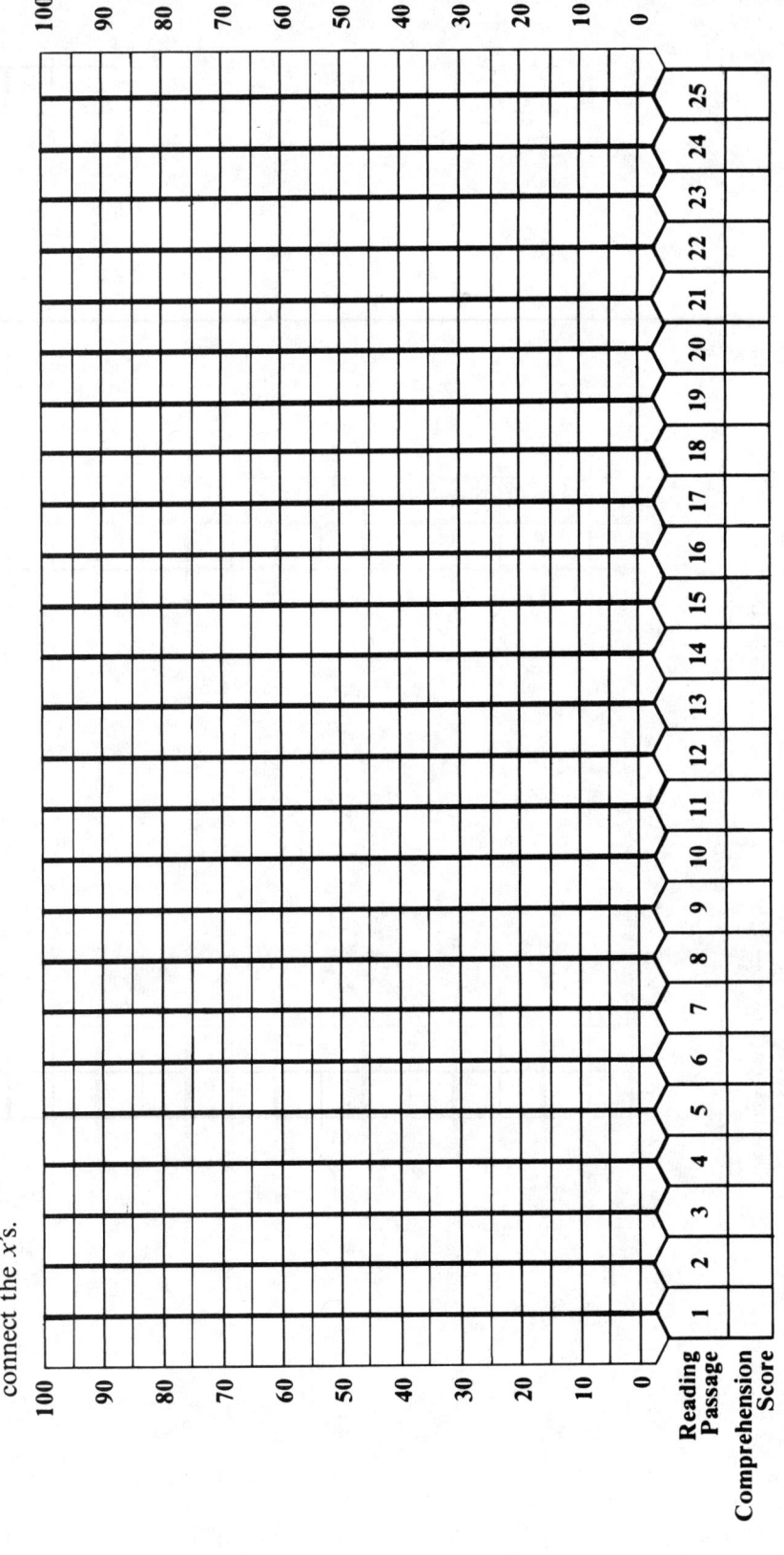

103

**Classroom
Management
System**

Essential Skills Series

Classroom Management System
(For Teacher Correction)

To the Teacher

The Classroom Management System provides an easy and effective way to individualize instruction. It can be used by reading specialists as well as by regular classroom teachers. The management system is designed to be equally effective when used with a single student, a small group, or a full-size class.

The Classroom Management System provides ongoing assessment of student work for both you and your student. It shows not only the amount of work completed, but also the quality of the work.

It serves as a diagnostic tool by revealing patterns of errors at a glance. For example, if a student has difficulty identifying subject matter (question #1 in each set of questions throughout the *Essential Skills Series*), a pattern of errors will appear in the Subject Matter column of the Classroom Management System Record Sheet. This will enable you to focus on the specific skills needs of each student.

The Classroom Management System Record Sheet is on pages 108-109. Both pages may be duplicated and stapled together.

How to Use the Classroom Management System Record Sheet

Step 1: Have the student answer the questions for each *Essential Skills* passage under the appropriate question heading.

Passage	① Subject Matter	② Supporting Details	③ Conclusion	④ Clarifying Devices	⑤ Vocabulary in Context	⑥ Main Idea				Number Correct	Errors Corrected
						a	b	c	d		
1	d	c	a	b	d		N	D	M		

Step 2: Circle any incorrect answers and fill in the total number correct.

1	d	ⓒ	a	b	d		N	D	M	6	

Step 3: Have the student correct his or her incorrect answers.

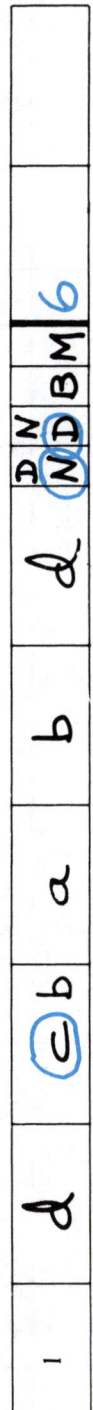

Step 4: Give assistance as needed and, if necessary, correct the student's adjusted answers.

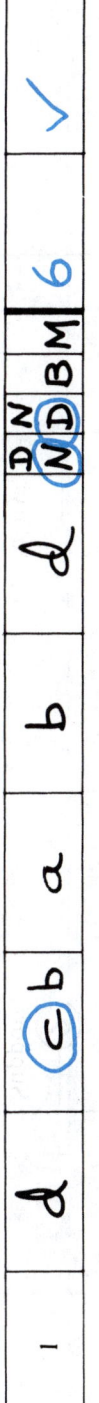

Step 5: Have the student go on to the next passage.

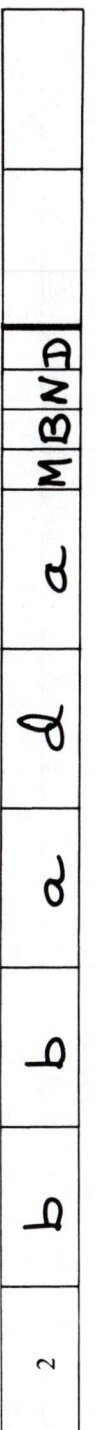

Step 6: Repeat Steps 1-4. If the class is large, it may be necessary to have students complete two or three passages before you correct them. This will slow the "traffic" at your desk.

Note: It is important for students to analyze and, to the extent possible, correct their own errors (Step 3).

Essential Skills Series

Classroom Management System Record Sheet
(For Teacher Correction)

Name _____

Teacher _____

Date _____

Book Number _____

To the Student: Write your answers in the spaces provided. (See the Example below.) Your teacher will circle any incorrect answers. Then go back over the questions and correct your mistakes.

Passage	① Subject Matter	② Supporting Details	③ Conclusion	④ Clarifying Devices	⑤ Vocabulary in Context	⑥ Main Idea a	b	c	d	Number Correct	Errors Corrected
Example	c	(b) a	d	a	c	a (b)	c	d			
1											
2											
3											
4											
5											
6											
7											
8											
9											
10											

Name _____ Book No. _____ Classroom Management System Record Sheet

Name	1	2	3	4	5	6							
11													
12													
13													
14													
15													
16													
17													
18													
19													
20													
21													
22													
23													
24													
25													

This record sheet may be duplicated for classroom use by teachers.
From *Essential Skills Series* by Walter Pauk, copyright © 1982 by Jamestown Publishers. Classroom Management System by Thomas F. Kelly, Ph.D.